AF324854

Vol. 2

Series on Biomaterials and Bioengineering

Life-Enhancing
PLASTICS

Plastics and Other Materials in
Medical Applications

Vol. 2
Series on Biomaterials and Bioengineering

Life-Enhancing PLASTICS

Plastics and Other Materials in Medical Applications

Anthony Holmes-Walker

BioInteractions Ltd, UK

Imperial College Press

Published by

Imperial College Press
57 Shelton Street
Covent Garden
London WC2H 9HE

Distributed by

World Scientific Publishing Co. Pte. Ltd.
5 Toh Tuck Link, Singapore 596224
USA office: Suite 202, 1060 Main Street, River Edge, NJ 07661
UK office: 57 Shelton Street, Covent Garden, London WC2H 9HE

British Library Cataloguing-in-Publication Data
A catalogue record for this book is available from the British Library.

LIFE-ENHANCING PLASTICS: PLASTICS AND OTHER MATERIALS IN MEDICAL APPLICATIONS
Series on Biomaterials and Bioengineering — Vol. 2
Copyright © 2004 by Imperial College Press

ISBN 1-86094-462-0

Printed by FuIsland Offset Printing (S) Pte Ltd, Singapore

ACKNOWLEDGEMENTS

I should like to acknowledge the very considerable help given in the preparation of this book, by a large number of people who have been generous in their efforts to assist in such tasks as: reading the manuscript, discussing the format and content of the work, as well as sharing their ideas and original research.

The most noteworthy are: Professors Richard and Andrew Batchelor, Professor Richard Beard, Mr Michael Brough, Professor Gianni Angelini, Mr Nicholas Beechey-Newman, Dr Martin Bryant, Dr Michael Boyes, Professor Kevin Warwick, Mr John Hobby, Mr Paul Taylor, Mr John Kirkup, the late Miss Alma West, Ms Sue Ellis, Mr Ken Jones, Mr Noel James, Mr Tony Anson, and particularly my wife Marie-Anne, as well as my daughters Antonia and Katharine for their constant encouragement.

I am also grateful to the many individuals and organisations who have allowed me to reproduce illustrations of their products and research, and I have acknowledged their help in the text.

Materials, both natural and synthetic, have been used for thousands of years in an attempt to cure, or at least alleviate, the diseases and misfortunes which affect the functioning of the human body.

The range of solutions is enormous: from simple contact applications; such as plastic lenses for the eye, through wound closure methods—adhesives. sutures and staples—to the use of permanently implanted devices; including hip replacements and cardiac pacemakers.

The purpose of this book is to enable people without specialist knowledge to gain an understanding of the ways in which materials in general, and plastics in particular, can be used to enhance the quality of life of those needing medical treatment or surgical intervention.

My approach to the subject has been that of the scientist and engineer—my own background—and in this I am conscious of the very real difference in attitude between the medical practitioner and the "rest of us". Although the medical student's syllabus contains a scientific element, the emphasis gradually veers, quite properly, towards less quantifiable aspects: the make up of the human body and how it copes with congenital abnormalities, the onset of age, disease and infirmity, not to mention the repair of all kinds of damage along the way. There is now, fortunately, an increased awareness of the contribution which machines and modern technology can make to achieve these objectives, and we shall see later how highly sophisticated "automated" techniques—such as robotics—are being used in the operating theatre. The use of multidisciplinary teams, in both research and treatment, is also now becoming commonplace. However, although the understanding and appreciation are there, the standpoint remains—and has to remain—different.

As we shall see the number of parts of the human body which can be repaired or replaced is truly remarkable; especially since many of the replacement parts are marvels of miniaturisation, reliability and sophistication. So many parts of the body can be replaced by mechanical alternatives that the "Bionic Man", beloved of fiction writers, is almost here. In order, therefore, to explore the use of materials in the human body, I have considered it appropriate to deal in some detail with the ways in which the body reacts to the introduction of hostile components, and how it handles them. I have also dealt with the important challenge of how the scientist, the engineer and the doctor are together able to minimise the adverse consequences of this intrusion. Before dealing with these subjects, however, I felt it would be useful for me to provide a fairly brief survey—in general terms—of the development of surgical techniques, together with some pointers to the future. In this latter context, it must be emphasised here, as I have done elsewhere, that the advance of modern technology is so great, especially in the field of robotics, minimally invasive surgery, and miniaturisation, that procedures which seemed impossibly far-fetched when I started researching this book three years ago, are now becoming accepted methods of surgical intervention.

Although, in a book of this nature it has been necessary to introduce a fair degree of scientific detail, I hope that the treatment will make it of value and interest, not only to those who later intend to specialise in the medical, engineering or scientific fields, but also to more general readers, such as those taking A-levels, MBA students &c., as well as to anyone who wishes to learn something about the use of materials in medical applications.

CONTENTS

Chapter 1
Surgical Techniques

1.1. Introduction

Whilst the main thrust of this book is on the ways in which materials, especially plastics, can be used to solve problems in surgery and medicine, I felt it would be valuable—particularly for those readers without a medical background—to provide a general overview of the principal surgical procedures, and the ways in which surgeons have developed and improved their art.

It will then be possible to discuss specific techniques in later chapters, with particular reference to the materials used, and their contribution to the different procedures. Inevitably, in the space available and for this type of book, I can only attempt to cover this vast subject in very general terms. Also, for the same reasons, although pretty well every organ in the human body has been operated upon, I have confined myself to the more familiar areas of surgery, and for those where plastics and other man-made materials play an important part. Although I have included, in this chapter, as in others, references in the text, I have also at the end of the book—for the reader who wishes to study further—added a selection of more specialised sources under "further reading". Some of these are books and papers, and others are Internet references.

I shall be covering the topics against a backdrop of the problems which have had to be overcome, together with the developments which have made advances possible, and will give some pointers to the ways in which progress might be achieved in the future. Also, in order to avoid making this chapter inordinately long, I have drawn a rather artificial line under what may be called "normal surgery", even if carried out "in miniature". The more innovative techniques, including minimal access surgery, the use of robotics and computer modelling, will be dealt with in a later chapter.

1.2. Historical Perspective

In the middle ages physicians considered that, although sometimes necessary, surgery—usually limited to blood letting, the removal of external growths, or the repair of superficial damage—was beneath their notice, and should be left to the "manual labourers" of the craft.

As a result, there developed the barber surgeon, the wound surgeon and the surgeon apothecary. Some of these rather quaint titles have survived to the present day, although their holders are invariably highly qualified professionals. Examples include the Serjeant Surgeon to the Queen and the Apothecary to the Household of

Windsor. The American armed forces, and the US Government, also have a Surgeon General.

By the 18th century, with increasing knowledge of anatomy, the successful amputation of legs and arms, the excision of tumours on, or just below, the skin surface, and the removal of stones from the bladder, led to a growing respect for surgery, and even the surgeon himself!

In the early 19th century surgeons were beginning to become more adventurous, but were hampered in their enthusiasm by the pain suffered by the patient during these operations. One result of this limitation was that surgeons tended to speed up their operative procedures so as to complete as much as possible before the patient could stand the pain and stress no longer! It took almost a hundred years, and the introduction of really effective anaesthetics, before surgeons learned to slow down.

This more leisurely approach also made it possible to introduce new techniques. Basic procedures were refined: instead of cutting in any direction to save time, surgeons learned to cut parallel to the skin's natural crevices and folds. This procedure—pioneered by Carl von Langer (1819–1877), professor of anatomy in Vienna—had the twofold result of reducing the tendency for the wound to pull open against the stitches, and the production of less unsightly scars. Fig. 1.1 shows an operation being performed in about 1900.

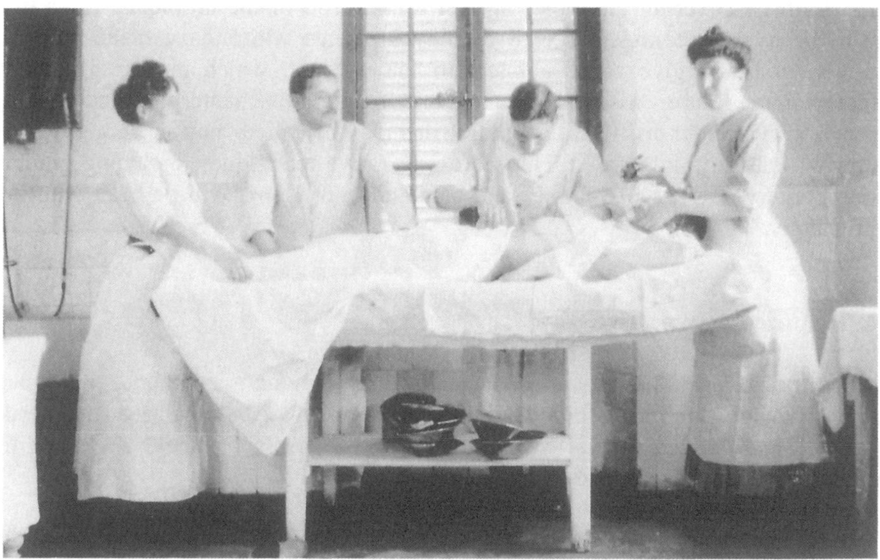

Figure 1.1   A French surgeon operating in about 1900. Though clean, the theatre is not sterile. (Courtesy Roger-Viollet, Paris)

1.2.1. The Discovery of Anaesthesia

As early as 1799, the chemist Sir Humphrey Davy (1778–1829) suggested that nitrous oxide could be used as an analgesic and general anaesthetic in surgical operations, but it was not until 1844 that Horace Wells (1815–1848) used nitrous oxide to produce anaesthesia during dental extractions, and, in 1846, he confirmed the findings in a public demonstration. At about the same time William T G Morton (1819–1868) showed that the inhalation of ether vapour produced insensibility to pain.

The terms "anaesthesia" and "anaesthetic" were first suggested in 1846, after Wells' and Morton's successful demonstrations, by the American physician, poet and humourist Oliver Wendell Holmes (1809–1894). It should be noted here that there is a difference between anaesthesia and "analgesia", both often used erroneously to mean the same thing. Anaesthesia, whether it affects part or all of the body, is brought about in such a manner that the patient is not conscious of any sensation in the anaesthetised part of the body. Analgesia, on the other hand, as its name suggests, offers pain relief without necessarily having a change in the level of consciousness

In the 1920s and 1930s several new gases were added to the list, and were later joined by drugs such as pentothal, which could be injected intravenously. Though these general anaesthetics were effective, either alone or in combination, there remained one main area of difficulty: how to make the patient's muscles relax when performing certain operations, such as abdominal surgery, without the necessity for very high drug doses. The answer lay in a poison from the rain forests of South America—curare. As long ago as 1811, the English physiologist and surgeon Sir Benjamin Brodie (1783–1862), had recognised the beneficial properties of curare, and was the first to show that artificial respiration could maintain life in curarised animals. The drug was subsequently used with some success in the American Civil War.

Much later, in 1952, two Canadian physicians, Harold Griffith and Enid Johnson in Montreal, discovered that curare administered during an abdominal operation, allowed the amount of anaesthetic required to be greatly reduced, because the patient's muscles became completely relaxed. This discovery, although making surgery easier, brought its own problems in that it became necessary for the anaesthetist to take over the functioning of the patient's lungs.

After the discovery of these basic techniques, it became customary to tailor the type of anaesthesia to the needs of the patient and the nature of the operation, and for certain drugs to be administered some two hours before the operation. This "premedication" (or "premed") may contain an analgesic, together with an anxiolytic drug, to relieve pain and anxiety, and to reduce the dose of general anaesthetic required to produce unconsciousness.

General anaesthesia is usually induced by the intravenous injection of a drug such as propofol, and maintained by the inhalation of the vapour of a volatile liquid: eg isoflurane, or a gas such as nitrous oxide mixed with oxygen It is arguable that one of the factors which has most influenced the potential of surgeons is the use of postoperative analgesia, which allows the patient to recover peacefully after the operation.

1.2.2. Combating Infection

Whenever the skin is broken, whether by an operation or by injury, the body's natural barrier to infection is breached, allowing the entry of bacteria which can spread and cause infection. The prevention and control of infection is, therefore, an important factor in surgical procedures. A considerable reduction in the spread of infection can be achieved by simply imposing the disciplines of washing the hands, wearing clean operating gowns, using sterile instruments and the provision of near-sterile operating theatres. The gauze face-mask was introduced in Europe as a means of preventing airborne infection at about the beginning of the 20th century.

Other developments, such as the "antisepsis" of Joseph Lister (1827–1912), which involved the use of chemical agents for killing bacteria, and the employment of "asepsis"—the use of heat for sterilisation—further reduced the risk of serious infection.

The pioneering work of Florence Nightingale (1820–1910), beginning with the elimination of the filth and insanitary conditions of the military hospitals in the Crimea (1854), and the establishment of a training school for nurses in St. Thomas's Hospital, London, in 1860, laid the foundations for modern standards of cleanliness and hygiene in both military and civilian hospitals, and in the whole arena of public health.

Ironically enough, the simple fact of the introduction of rubber gloves—now taken for granted, and used almost universally by any professional person (doctors, paramedics, nurses, dentists, vets, the police and social workers) against the risk of infection—occurred by chance in 1906. The American surgeon William Halstead, when preparing for an operation, found that one of the theatre nurses (later to become his wife) complained that the disinfectants then in use caused her to have an allergic reaction on the skin of her hands. Halstead suggested the gloves, and later it was discovered their use, by all members of the team, considerably reduced the rates of accidental infection.

1.2.3. Shock

One of the most common after-effects of any serious injury is shock. Used in the medical sense, the term "shock" refers to a potentially catastrophic reduction in blood pressure—brought about either by extensive bleeding, or through sudden failure of the circulatory system. Left untreated, shock can be fatal, since, in severe cases, the decreased interchange of the gases, salts and proteins carried by the blood, causes profound changes in the function of the body's organs and tissues.

Over 150 years ago it was found that saline injections could sometimes reduce the effects of shock. It was not, however, until the 1930s that intravenous injections of saline solutions became the routine method of treatment on the spot. The most obvious way to replace lost blood, the transfusion of whole blood, had been attempted over hundreds of years, often with fatal results. Fig. 1.2 shows a procedure, demonstrated at Guy's Hospital in London by James Blundell (1790–1877), for transfusing whole blood. Blood is allowed to fall into a warmed funnel, from which it flows into the recipient's vein.

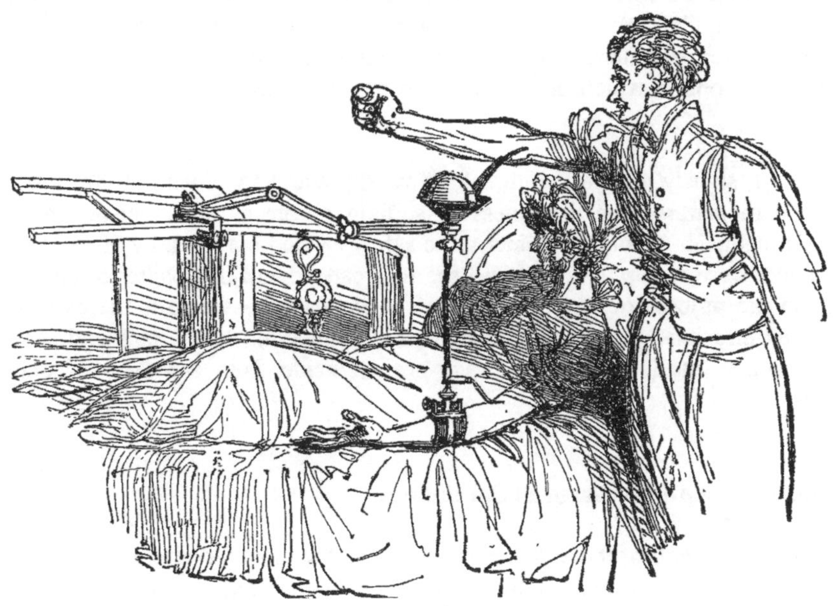

Figure 1.2 James Blundell's transfusion set-up (Courtesy The Lancet)

In 1900 the Austrian scientist Karl Landsteiner (1868–1943) who, in 1930 won the Nobel prize for medicine, observed that when blood samples taken from several different people were mixed with serum from the others (serum is that part of the blood remaining after removal of all cellular elements), some of the mixtures stayed clear while others formed clumps of the red cells (agglutination).

Landsteiner's next task was to explain the phenomenon. He found that some people's red blood cells carried a particular surface protein, which he called A, while others carried a different one, which he called B. Some people have both, others have one, while some have neither. The four combinations: A, B, AB and O; described the four blood groups. He also found that the clear serum could contain two other proteins, called anti-A and anti-B, which were able to react with the surface proteins to cause agglutination.

One of the factors causing blood to clot is temperature, so—to prevent clotting—blood was transfused directly from one person to another (see Fig. 1.2). This method, although somewhat inconvenient, ensured not only that the blood was at the right temperature, but also avoided the possibility of accidental infection. It was also found that, provided the blood groups matched, person–to–person transfusion could be carried out from a succession of donors, and I am aware of a case in Oakland, California, when a woman received transfusions from three donors at the birth of her daughter in 1928. However, a better method was clearly required, and preferably one in which the blood could be stored before being transfused into the recipient.

In 1914, shortly after the outbreak of World War I, A Hustin (1882–1967) of Belgium demonstrated the usefulness of sodium citrate as an anticoagulant; thus enabling transfusion from a container to be safely carried out; and, by 1935, the first blood banks were set up. As we shall see in greater detail in Chapter 5, the use of plastics in the process of blood transfusion is extensive—as also is the case of all intravenous infusion—in that the cannulae, the connecting tubes, taps and sockets, and the sachets used for blood storage are all made from a variety of plastics materials.

1.3. Under the Knife — Surgical Specialities

Whilst the second half of the 20th century has seen the most far-reaching advances in surgical techniques, and some of these will be discussed later, it may come as quite a surprise to discover how long ago surgeons were practising, and perfecting, some extremely sophisticated procedures. So as to preserve some kind of order, I shall start with the head, and then progress downwards to the chest and abdomen, and thence to the arms and lower limbs. I shall also concentrate on the procedures which have evolved by what may be described as "open" surgery, before turning to the more recent and sophisticated techniques of micro, and minimal access surgery.

1.3.1. Neurosurgery — The Brain

In most cases neurosurgery involves cutting through the skull, either to relieve pressure or to perform an operation on a specific site. While surgeons have been drilling through the skull for hundreds of years (see Chapter 9), and had—with some success—treated abscesses and tumours on the outer surface of the brain, entry into the brain itself required a great deal of knowledge and dexterity, much of which was achieved by trial and error.

A distinguished pioneer in this field was the American surgeon Harvey Cushing (1869–1939). He was professor of surgery at Harvard University from 1912 and, owing to his ability and attention to detail, the death rate during brain surgery dropped from over 30% to as little as 5%.

Neurosurgery has developed into a highly sophisticated branch of the art; and—in order to avoid damage to the delicate nerve tissue—it is necessary not only to use surgical techniques in which the margin of error is virtually nil, but also to be able to locate the site of the operation, be it blood clot or tumour, with the utmost precision. These exacting requirements are achieved by the following procedures: the head is immobilised by attaching the skull, by means of pins or screws, to a mechanical arm which is rigidly attached to the operating table. Fig. 1.3 shows such a device.

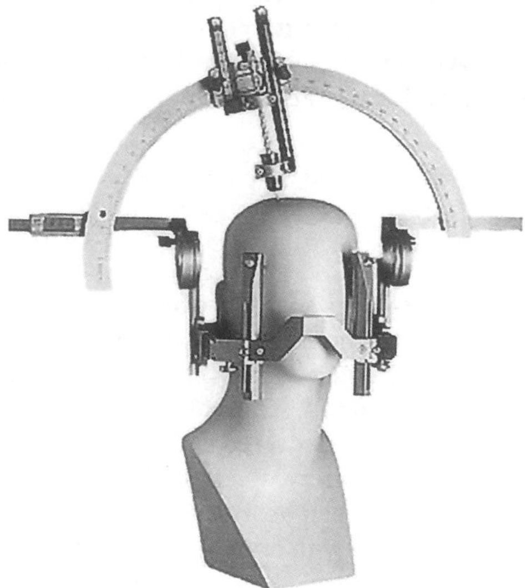

Figure 1.3 Application of a frame to stabilise the patient's head during neurosurgery. (Courtesy The Gamma Knife Center, West Palm Beach, Florida).

The surgeon can then be guided to the right spot by a combination of methods: the use of a low-powered microscope, and a technique known as "stereotaxy". In this the patient's head is surrounded by a metal cage, which acts like a grid for reference purposes. The information obtained by this means is fed into a computer, the output from which enables the instruments to reach the target with minimal damage to the surrounding tissue.

Whilst microscopes and stereotaxy can help to guide the surgeon, it must be remembered that using the former does restrict the area which can be seen, as well as distorting the depth of focus. The effect, and possible damage caused by the high intensity lighting required to illuminate the field must also be appreciated.

A more sophisticated version of stereotaxy makes use of a system which provides a three-dimensional image of the brain. The location of the tumour or clot may be determined both before and during the operation by the use of X-rays, computer tomography, screening and magnetic resonance imaging. The images generated by these means are often displayed on a screen in the operating theatre (or any other remote station) to assist the surgical team during the operation.

I have so far mentioned only the excision of tumours and blood clots. However, there are other conditions, including the treatment of a variety of malfunctions of the arteries and veins (aneurysms &c.), neuralgia; as well as the removal of parts of the brain itself, which can be carried out by "gamma knife surgery" (stereotaxic radiosurgery)(1). This extremely powerful tool uses a large number of highly focussed gamma rays. Its advantages include the fact that recovery is rapid, since there is no actual incision, and the whole operation is carried out under local anaesthetic.

1.3.2. Vascular Surgery

In 1894 Alexis Carrel (1873–1944), a surgeon working in Lyon, saw the French President—Marie-Francois Carnot—die from stab wounds because nobody was able to join the two halves of a severed artery. The problem was that the severed ends, not being filled with blood, had collapsed. Carrel experimented for eight years until he developed a method whereby the two severed ends could be joined together using a trio of stitches. Each section of the artery was provided with three loops of stitches (Fig. 1.4). When the stitches were pulled apart simultaneously, each end opened up into a triangle, making it easier to join with normal surgical stitches .

However, even this elegant solution had its drawbacks. The internal surface of a healthy undamaged blood vessel offers no impediment to the smooth passage of the blood. The presence of a stitch can lead to the formation of a clot (thrombus), which

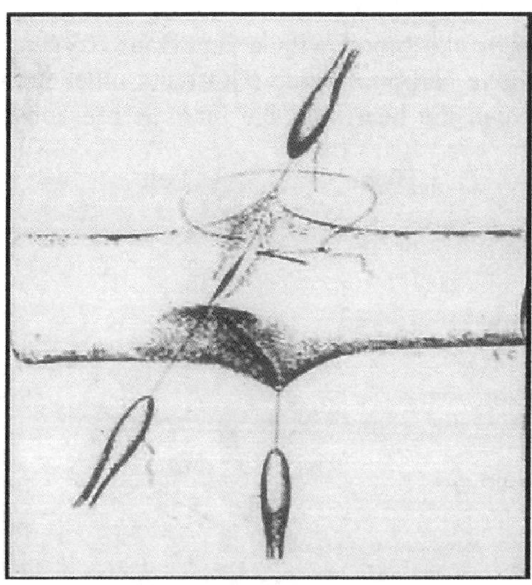

Figure 1.4 Alexis Carrel's procedure for suturing a collapsed artery or vein

could cause a blockage, and which, if it became detached (forming an embolus), could travel to the lungs or brain with potentially fatal results. Carrel persisted in his attempts to overcome this problem and, in 1902, perfected a procedure whereby each severed end was rolled back upon itself to form a short collar, which could then be joined together without any of the stitches penetrating the inner wall of the vessel itself. It must be remembered that in those days, as well as the techniques, the implements and materials available were limited: curved needles had not yet appeared, and horsehair was commonly used for suturing. Silk only became popular largely as a result of Carrel's own work.

For his work on the suturing of blood vessels, which laid the foundations for all major surgical procedures, including organ transplantation, Carrel was awarded the Nobel prize for physiology and medicine in 1912.

1.3.3. Operating on the Lungs and Heart

As their functions are so closely interconnected, it is convenient to treat the lungs and heart as a single complex unit. However, since they handle two very different substances, air and blood, we can deal with their surgery separately.

1.3.4. The Lungs

The principal function of the lungs—which lie on both sides of the heart—is, in simple terms, to provide the blood with a supply of oxygen from the air through inhalation, and to remove carbon dioxide (CO_2) and other impurities by exhalation. The relationship between the heart and the lungs is presented diagrammatically in Fig. 1.5.

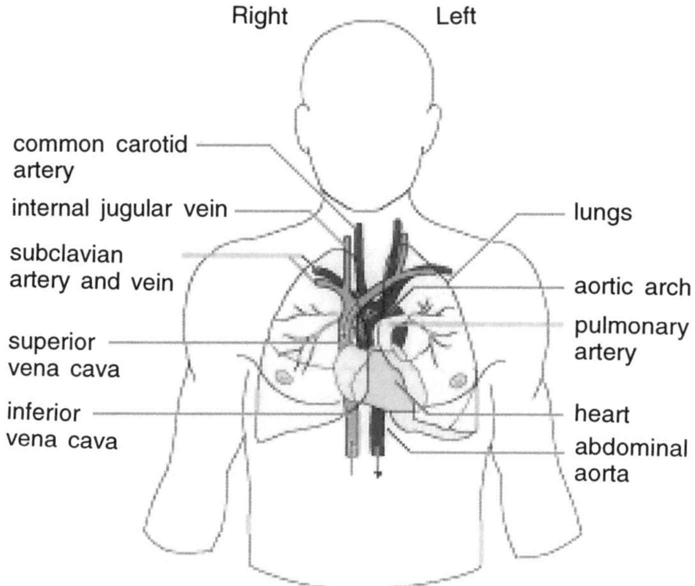

Figure 1.5 The relationship between the lungs and heart

The lungs themselves are surrounded by a sac-like membrane, and the whole assembly is contained in the space between the diaphragm and the rib-cage. Any movement of either of these two boundaries will alter the volume of the lungs. When the lungs are expanded, air enters into a system of narrowing passages which terminate in small sacs called alveoli. Tiny blood vessels surround each of the 300 million alveoli, and the oxygen—which moves across the walls of the sacs—is transported by these veins back to the heart, and thence to the entire body. Fig. 1.6 gives a diagrammatic view of the trachea and bronchi, together with the alveoli and blood vessels.

As the air passes through, it is warmed and humidified, and the dust and other debris removed. Once in contact with the alveolar surface, oxygen from the inhaled air is exchanged with the carbon dioxide suspended in the blood, and then the CO_2 laden gas is exhaled.

1.3.5. Surgery on the Lungs

When, in the 19th century, surgeons attempted to operate on the chest they encountered the problem of air pressure. The lungs, having little independent muscle power, expand and contract with the movements of the chest. The lungs are surrounded by a narrow space called the pleural cavity, which is filled with a lubricating fluid. In normal breathing the pressure in this space is lower than atmospheric pressure, and this keeps the lungs flexed outwards. If, during surgery, the cavity wall is punctured, air can enter and the lungs collapse.

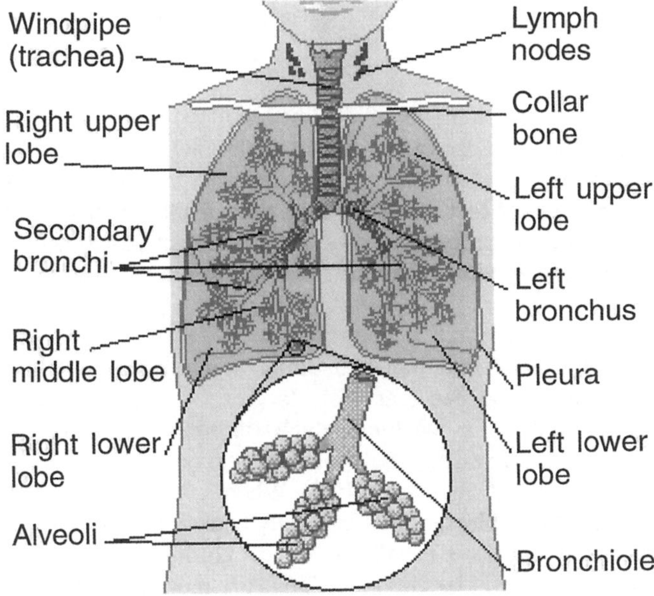

Figure 1.6 The lungs, showing the trachea, bronchi, the alveoli, and the blood vessels

In the early 1900s Ernst Sauerbruch (1875–1951), from Breslau, overcame the problem by encasing the patient, from the neck downwards, in an airtight chamber—which was kept at a pressure below that of the air outside—thus allowing the patient's lungs to function normally. Sauerbruch and his team worked inside the chamber. Although the procedure worked well, it was not popular with other surgeons and, by the end of World War I, it was replaced by a much simpler method: a tube fitted with an inflatable silicone rubber collar, which was inserted into the windpipe. As well as providing an airtight seal, the tube could be used for anaesthetic purposes, in addition to ventilating patients who were paralysed. Care had to be taken, however, to ensure that the seal was not so tight as to damage the internal surface of the windpipe.

Oddly enough, in the 1960s, a reverse adaptation of Sauerbruch's "tent" was used—this time under elevated pressure—to increase the diffusion rate of oxygen through the lungs, so that surgeons could 'buy' time to operate on "blue babies", whose condition arose from a lack of oxygen in the blood supply.

It is impossible to discuss the lungs without mentioning lung cancer. As early as 1912 some doctors believed that smoking tobacco and cancer of the lungs were interrelated, but were unable to establish the link. It was not until the early 1950s that proof began to emerge of a positive link between smoking and lung cancer. These results came from the work, published in 1950, of Ernst Wynder and Evarts Graham in the USA, and (in 1954) by Sir Richard Doll and Bradford Hill in the United Kingdom.

At the time the only method of dealing with the disease was to remove the affected tissue, and later to use radiation and chemotherapy. The alternative, a lung transplant, had been considered for some time and the first such operation was performed in 1964. Other candidates for lung transplantation include those suffering from advanced fibrotic lung diseases, who are dependent on oxygen therapy. Also, possible cases are those with pulmonary vascular disease, and chronic pulmonary infections.

In the case of a single lung transplantation, which is performed under a general anaesthetic, it is not always necessary for blood to be diverted from the lungs and heart (on "bypass") using a machine which removes carbon dioxide and other impurities, as well as providing the blood with oxygen. Instead, very careful management of the blood-flow may suffice. When a double lung transplantation is involved, however, the implantation is generally carried out as two separate entities, and cardiopulmonary bypass is usually required. During the operation the patient's lung, or lungs, are removed and the donor lungs are then stitched into place. At the end of the operation, drainage tubes are inserted into the chest area so as to evacuate accumulated fluid, blood and air.

1.3.6. The Heart

The human heart is essentially a pump comprising two separate operating systems, one on each side of the organ. The right side (as viewed from the front) receives de-oxygenated (dark red) blood from the veins and pumps it into the lungs, where it becomes oxygenated. This oxygenated (bright red) blood from the lungs travels to the left half of the heart, and is then pumped to the head, trunk and limbs of the body. The major muscular pumping chambers are known as the ventricles, and both operate at the same time. Fig. 1.7 shows a layout of the heart and its more important components.

Each ventricle is fed from its atrium—the smaller, bell-shaped, minor pumping chamber—situated between the blood vessel and the ventricle. The output of the ventricle is proportional to the pressure in the atrium which supplies it, and the level of output is determined by the requirements of the body at the time. Under normal relaxed conditions, the heart delivers about 80 ml of blood into the lung capillaries with each beat. During intense physical activity, however, the blood throughput can rise fourfold; from an average 5 litres per minute to over 20. In order to keep the body functioning harmoniously, the pressure gradients between the ventricles, the capillaries they feed, and the venous return to the atria are particularly important.

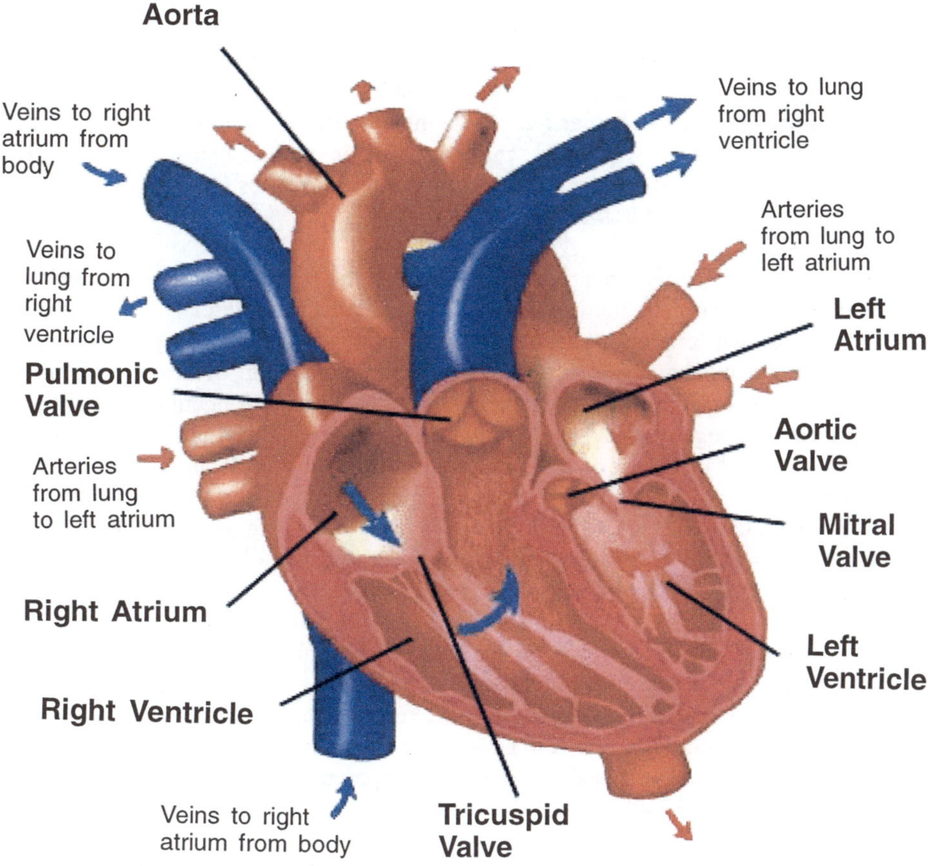

Figure 1.7 The human heart showing blood circulation paths

Although the blood has to travel through a considerable network of arteries, veins and capillaries during its journey round the body, there are so many pathways that very little resistance is offered to its passage. In fact, the blood that enters the right ventricle is already returning to the left atrium by the time of the next heartbeat (although , because of the special geography of the organ, this is not the case of the left ventricle and right atrium).

1.3.7. Heart Surgery

The American surgeon John Gibbon (1903–1973) developed, in 1952, the first heart-lung machine, which allowed the patient's blood to be removed from the body and oxygenated mechanically. This, and the use of induced hypothermia, made it possible for the heart to be stopped for more than an hour. This meant that relatively ambitious operations could be carried out on the heart itself and, by the 1960s, many patients had undergone successful valve repairs or replacements, and the first attempts were being made to correct blocked coronary arteries by using sections of vein taken from elsewhere in the body.

In 1962, the American heart surgeon James Hardy (1919–2003) performed the first heart transplant on a human patient. Medically and ethically it was not a success. Hardy was attempting to transplant a healthy heart from a donor who was on a life-support machine, and who seemed to be on the point of death. When the time came to perform the operation, the donor's heart was still beating strongly and he was, therefore, legally still alive. In his desire to keep the failing recipient alive, Hardy transplanted the heart of a chimpanzee. Although the donated heart worked well for a time, it proved to be too small—despite the assistance of pacemakers—to pump blood round the much larger human body, and the patient died shortly afterwards. In spite of the ensuing indignation over the ethical considerations, Hardy had demonstrated that heart transplantation was technically feasible.

As everyone knows by now, on the 2nd of December 1967, the world's first successful human heart transplant was performed by Dr Christian Barnard (1922–2001) on Louis Washkansky at the Groote Schuur Hospital in Capetown, South Africa. The donor was a young woman pedestrian knocked down by a lorry. Although her heart was still beating, there was apparently no hope of recovery, and she was certified as clinically dead.

Unfortunately Washkansky only survived for 18 days before dying of a lung infection, but the race was on; heart transplant operations followed at an alarming rate. Four days later, Adrian Kantrowitz (1918–   ) carried out a heart transplant on a young child in New York, and—a month later, also in the USA—Norman Shumway (1923–   ) operated on a 57 year old man. Both patients died, the child within hours and the man 15 days later. In January 1968, Barnard performed his second transplant, and the patient lived for 18 months, restoring, to some extent, public confidence in this risky and very costly procedure.

By the end of 1968 more than 100 transplants had been carried out, but few of the patients survived, because the organ was "foreign" to the recipient and, therefore, was "rejected". It was not until the development of effective immunosuppressive drugs that the problems of tissue rejection were dramatically reduced, and all types of transplant patients (heart, lungs, heart/lungs, liver and kidney) had a good expectation of life after the operation.

The replacement of a diseased human heart by a donor organ, although a highly complex and time-consuming operation, is a process which is well understood and capable of being carried out successfully. Therefore, I propose—having regard to the scope of this book—to deal only briefly with the transplantation procedure itself. For the same reason, it is sensible to consider—in outline only—some other surgical procedures on and close to the heart.

1.3.8. The Heart Transplant Operation

During the operation, the patient's blood is diverted from the heart and lungs ("on bypass") and pumped back into the body after removing carbon dioxide (a waste product) and replacing it with the oxygen needed by the body tissues. The surgical team then removes the heart, except for the back walls of the atria. The donor heart, after removal from the donor, is cooled, so that it can survive for a while unattached to the blood circulation. The backs of the donor heart atria are then opened, and the organ is sewn into place. The blood vessels are then connected, and the blood is allowed to flow through the new heart and the lungs. As the heart warms up, it normally begins beating, although it is sometimes necessary to "kick-start" it with an electrical shock. After the surgeons have checked all the blood vessels for leaks, the patient can be removed from the heart-lung machine, and the process of closing the chest wall begins.

1.3.9. Heart/Lung Transplantation

A transplant of both organs is usually appropriate when the patient is likely to die from end-stage lung disease that also involves the heart. Such a condition includes severe pulmonary hypertension, a large increase in blood pressure in the vessels of the lungs that limits blood flow and delivery of oxygen to the rest of the body, as well as certain birth defects of the heart, which may lead to acquired pulmonary hypertension.

The combined heart and double lung transplantation, which was first performed in 1981, is a technically demanding operation, which commonly takes from 6 to 8 hours to complete. The donor operation involves removing the heart and lungs combined together, while the recipient's lungs and heart are removed separately. During the operation, the donor's and recipient's main airway (the trachea), the main artery (the aorta) and the upper chamber on the right side of the heart (the right atrium) are joined together. The operation is lengthy because special care has to be taken both to control bleeding and also to preserve vital nerves

After the operation, heart/lung recipients are vulnerable to infection, because—as with lung and heart transplants—the lungs are in direct contact with the environment. They have to be checked regularly for signs of lung rejection, using a fibre-optic bronchoscope. Fortunately, under normal circumstances, rejection of the new heart is relatively rare, so regular tissue examinations (heart biopsies) are not usually required.

1.3.10. Other Thoracic Surgery

We have so far dealt with a number of forms of thoracic surgery involving the lungs and heart. However, there are other procedures, and we should at least consider the most important.

It is convenient to subdivide the large field of thoracic surgery into two main types:

* General – which deals with disorders of the lungs and oesophagus
* Cardiothoracic – which encompasses disorders of the heart and pericardium.

Although, as mentioned, there are several conditions which can indicate the need for surgery within the chest cavity, it will be sufficient to discuss one of the more significant; the treatment of an aneurysm.

An aortic aneurysm is a dilation of the aorta, the primary artery of the body that carries blood from the heart to the brain and other vital organs, including the upper and lower extremities. The principal risk of an aneurysm is that it could rupture, with potentially fatal results. Aortic aneurysms may occur either in the chest (thoracic) or the abdomen (abdominal). The risks do vary somewhat, however, since the average mortality following rupture of an abdominal aneurysm exceeds 75%, and that following a thoracoabdominal aneurysm reaches 95%. In the case of a thoracic aneurysm, the mortality falls to less than 5%. Before dealing with surgical repair of aneurysms specifically, I would like briefly to describe thoracic surgery in very general terms.

Thoracic surgery commonly involves opening the chest cavity, under general anaesthetic, by means of a large incision, beginning below the shoulder blade and extending in a curved arc under the arm, to the front of the chest. The muscles are also cut, and the ribs are spread with a retractor. More recently, a minimally invasive surgical technique has emerged—known as video-assisted thoracic surgery (VATS)— which uses a thoracic endoscope to allow the surgeon to view the chest cavity. To use this technique a lung is collapsed, and 3 or 4 small incisions, or access ports, are made to allow insertion of the endoscope. During the procedure the surgeon views the inside of the cavity on a video monitor. After the operation, the incisions are sealed with adhesive.

The repair of an abdominal aneurysm may now be carried out by an even less intrusive procedure, endovascular repair, which does not involve opening the chest or abdominal wall at all. Fig. 1.8 shows the treatment of an aortic aneurysm in which the endovascular repair procedure was used..

A fabric covered collapsible metal graft (an endovascular stent graft)—mounted in a carrier system terminating in a plastic sheath—is introduced into the femoral artery via a small incision in the groin. Using fluoroscopic guidance, the upper edge of the stent graft is positioned just below the renal (kidney) arteries. The plastic sheath is then retracted, which allows the device to expand into its predetermined shape. The smaller limb is located in the iliac artery. Another, smaller, device is inserted into the opposite femoral artery, to allow positioning of the shorter limb of the prosthesis.

(a)

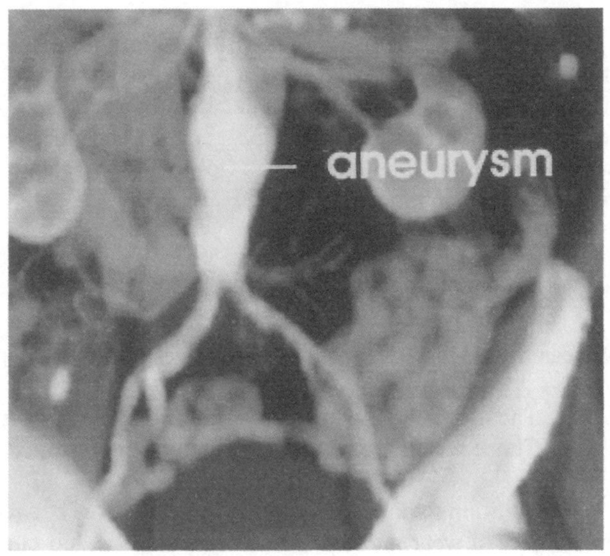

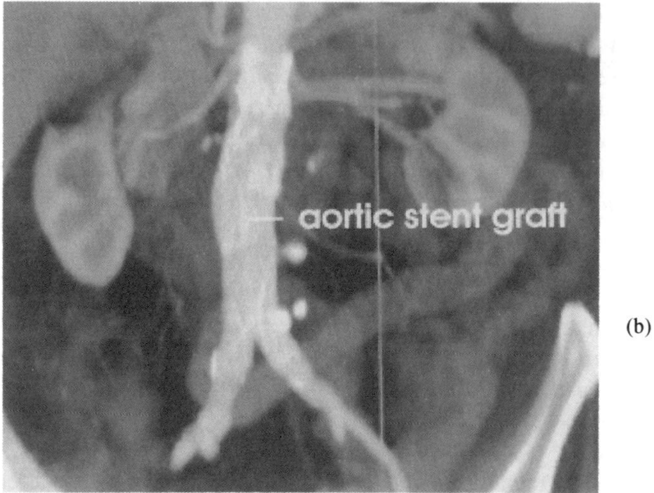

Figure 1.8 The repair of a thoracoabdominal aneurysm using an endovascular stent graft. (a) the condition before surgery, (b) the same patient one month after treatment

As in all operations, particularly those involving the arteries, such procedures carry risks. However, the mortality in endovascular repair is about half that when open surgery is used.

It must be recognised, though, that the more extensive aneurysms can only be treated by open surgery. Recent advances using the collaborative efforts of several disciplines, including: vascular and cardiac surgery, radiology, anaesthesia, perfusion technology, neurology, cardiology, genetics and microbiology, have minimised two serious complications sometimes following surgical procedures for aneurysmal repair—stroke and paraplegia..

1.3.11. The Repair of Defective Heart Valves

We can divide disorders of the heart valves into two categories:

* Those which develop as a result of disease or other damage
* Those which are inherent – usually from birth.

In addition to damage by infection, the valves between the chambers of the heart are subject to wear and tear. Each valve opens and closes some 30 million times a year—a staggering two thousand million (2 x 10^9) over an average lifetime! As a result, several things may happen, the valves may begin to leak, or may become narrowed (stenosis), and can start to obstruct the normal flow of blood. The valves which are most commonly affected are the mitral valve (between the two chambers on the left side of the heart), and the aortic valve (located at the outlet of the left ventricle).

In such cases the surgeon, depending on the severity of the damage, has two alternatives: to repair or to replace. Repair is generally carried out on mitral valves that are narrowed, or which tend to leak, but which are not otherwise badly damaged. When replacement of all or part of the valve is indicated, the surgeon has again two options: to use tissue valves, or mechanical replacement valves. Those in the latter category will be considered in more detail in Chapter 7, when we deal with long-term implanted materials.

Tissue valves fall into two categories: human tissue—which may be in the form of allografts (from another person), or autografts—where the valve is moved from one position to another within the same patient. Under certain circumstances, the performance of the valve may be improved by self-transplantation (re-siting the valve in or near to its original location)

It is also possible to use animal tissue valves (called heterografts or xenografts), where the valve tissue is generally taken from pigs. Non-valve tissue is also used, for example: bovine or cow pericardium (the membrane surrounding the heart).

An interesting technique was recently reported from Boston (2) where cells are seeded onto a porous valve-like bioabsorbable scaffold, and grown in an incubator under conditions similar to those inside the heart. After transplantation into sheep, the entire bioabsorbable scaffold was reported to have been resorbed and replaced with healthy cardiovascular tissue. A not entirely dissimilar idea has been put forward for "growing" artificial kidneys (3). I shall be referring to this technique again in Chapter 10, where we consider a range of exciting new methods for organ growth, replacement and repair.

Whatever corrective treatment is used, the surgeon has to approach the damaged valve via one of the atria, or major vessels that lead to the heart.

The most common of the congenital defects of the heart is the "hole in the heart"; a gap in the wall between the two upper, or lower, chambers. Some of these defects close naturally, others have to be repaired.   Open heart surgery, involving bypass, is currently used, although recently it has been found possible to pass through the blood vessels a small plastic "patch" (or plug) which is then implanted in the defect.

Although, as already pointed out, there will be other references for further reading later in the book, I thought it worth mentioning here an excellent book, recently produced by the Reader's Digest, and entitled "The Heart & Circulatory System" . This work treats the subject in a very comprehensive and readable fashion (4).

1.3.12. Liver Surgery

There is hardly a metabolic activity that does not involve either a substance secreted by the liver, or a substance whose concentration is not regulated by the liver. Some of its functions include manufacturing new body proteins and blood-clotting factors, producing bile that assists the breakdown of fatty foods, converting food into the chemicals necessary for life and growth, storing essential vitamins, minerals and carbohydrates, breaking down drugs and hormones, and removing toxins from the blood.

A healthy liver has a great capacity to repair itself, and can overcome most harmful things—infections or damage from alcohol or drugs. Sometimes, however, the damage is so severe that it causes rapid destruction of the liver cells, resulting in acute liver failure. In other cases the destruction is more gradual, leading to scarring. This scarring is irreversible, and leads to a condition called cirrhosis (chronic liver disease). Common causes of cirrhosis in adults are chronic hepatitis, sclerosis (replacement of normal tissue by a fibrous overgrowth), cholangitis (inflammation of the bile ducts), primary biliary cirrhosis and chronic alcohol abuse. A diagram of the liver and its relationship to the adjacent organs is shown in Fig. 1.9.

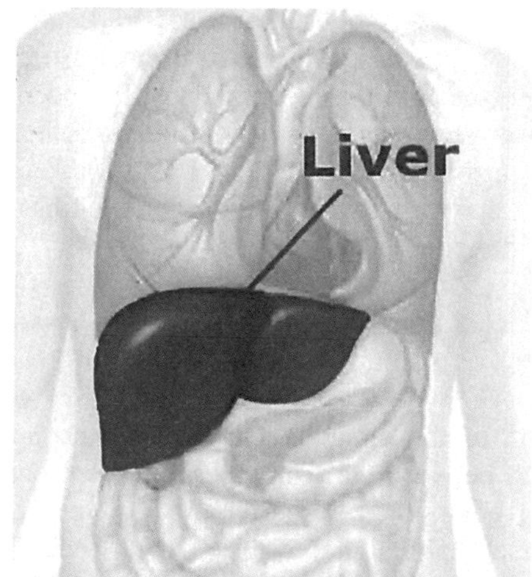

Figure 1.9 The liver and adjacent organs. (Courtesy University of Maryland Medicine, USA)

Although some of these disorders can be treated by the use of drugs, it is not possible, so far, to replace any of the liver's main functions by machines. Also, unlike the kidneys, there is only one liver in the body, and the more serious malfunctions have to be dealt with by transplantation. In the case of renal failure, it is possible to remove one kidney and survive satisfactorily on the remaining one. Where cancer of the liver is present, localised tumours can be excised. If it has spread, transplantation can be considered, but it is necessary to remove the whole liver.

In the case of liver transplantation, as with all attempts to implant either natural or artificial organs, we come up against rejection by the body's immune system. Patients undergoing such an operation will normally have to take immunosuppressive drugs for the rest of their lives. There have been cases, however, where patients who, after several years of faithful pill-taking, have stopped taking them—either because they simply forgot, became confused, or decided not to continue—and found, after a routine medical check-up, that the donated liver seemed to have become accepted by the body. This phenomenon seems to confirm the discoveries of Sir Peter Medawar (1915–1987), during and after World War II, on tissue rejection, which gained him the Nobel prize for Medicine in 1960, and which we shall discuss in Chapter 3.

Well aware of the problems resulting from tissue rejection, the American surgeon Thomas Starzl attempted the first human liver transplant in 1963. However, because of the liver's complicated blood supply system, success had to wait until 1967.

Nowadays, the transplant operation—which normally takes about 6-8 hours—involves the complete removal of the diseased liver, and its replacement with the donor organ. Entry into the abdominal cavity is through an inverted "Y" shaped incision, often called the "Mercedes Benz incision!" As is the case in other major abdominal surgery, and for operations on the heart and lungs, specialised equipment is used to assist the patient's breathing, monitor progress and recovery, and supply essential fluids and drugs.

1.3.13. Kidney Surgery

The function of the kidneys is to filter the blood in the body and produce urine. In so doing they cleanse the body of many drugs and toxins. The filtering unit (the glomerulus) processes the blood, and the filtrate drains into a sac (the Bowman capsule), and thence—via the renal tubules—into the bladder. The function of the tubules is, by absorption, to promote protein retention, and minimise water loss. The whole assembly is known as the "nephron". The kidneys also produce hormones and control the blood pressure. Fig. 1.10 gives a diagrammatic view of the kidney.

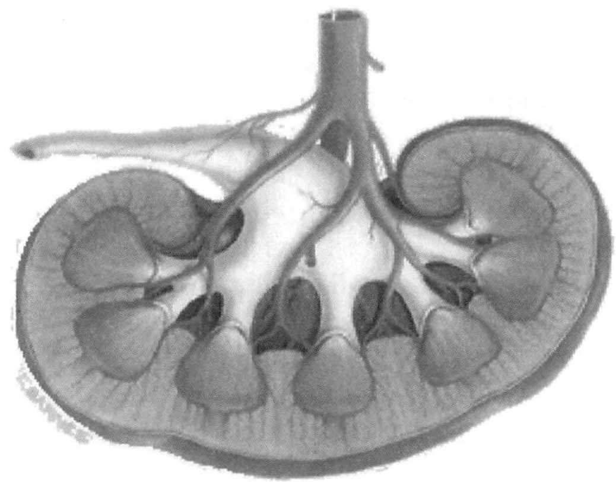

Figure 1.10 The human kidney. (Courtesy University of Maryland Medicine, USA)

Each kidney is supplied with blood by a large artery. This blood supply is essential, both for the health of the kidneys, and to allow them to perform their functions of cleansing and maintaining the blood.

Anything that leads to a sudden drop in blood flow to the kidneys can cause acute renal failure. When this happens, the normal functions of the kidneys can be affected or destroyed. Among the causes of acute renal failure are: a blockage of urine flow out of the kidneys and into the bladder, exposure to certain drugs, the effects of toxic substances, or—more rarely—the appearance of clotting in the renal vein.

Most disorders of the kidneys can usually be cured by the use of appropriate drug therapy, or alleviated by the use of long-term dialysis. When this is not possible, the alternative is the removal of one, or—depending on the nature and severity of the problem—both kidneys. The latter results in patients requiring renal dialysis or renal transplantation.

1.3.14. Kidney Transplantation

Kidney transplantation is performed on patients with chronic kidney failure, or end-stage renal disease (ESRD). The process involves surgically attaching a functioning kidney, or graft, from a brain-dead organ donor (cadaver transplant), or from a living donor, who may be either related or non-related to the recipient. Where the donor is related to the recipient, there is a considerably stronger chance of a successful biological match.

The surgical procedure of kidney removal (nephrectomy) from a living donor is performed under general anaesthetic. The incision is usually made on the side or front of the abdomen; the blood vessels connecting the kidney to the donor are clamped and severed, and the ureter is also clamped between the kidney and the bladder, and cut. The kidney—with the attached section of ureter—is then removed, the blood vessels and ureter tied off, and the incision closed. Much the same procedure is used to remove cadaver kidneys, although both are generally taken out at the same time, together with blood and cell samples for tissue typing. Once removed, the kidneys are placed on ice and flushed with a preservative solution until required for transplantation.

In the case of the recipient, antibiotics are administered to prevent infection, and a catheter placed in the bladder. The incision is made in the flank of the patient under general anaesthetic, and the donor kidney implanted above the pelvic bone, and below the existing non-functioning kidney, by suturing the renal artery and vein to the patient's iliac artery and vein (the vessels concerned with the transport of blood to and from the lower limbs and pelvic region). The ureter of the new organ is then attached directly to the bladder of the recipient. The diseased kidney may either be left in situ, or removed, depending on the nature of the disease and the circumstances surrounding the failure.

There is an extraordinary shortage of suitable kidneys for transplantation into patients with ESRD. For example, in 1998 in the United States, there were 42,570 registered patients awaiting transplants, and in the previous year only 8,606 cadaver kidneys were transplanted. Whilst the annual number of donor kidneys has remained stable at about 8,500 for the last five years, the renal transplant waiting list has grown by more than 13% per year over the same period. Also the average quality of cadaver donor kidneys has declined as the donor population has increased in age This being the case, there has been renewed interest in kidney transplants from living donors.. However, although the operation is entirely safe, living donor nephrectomy does require a 20–25 cm incision.

Recent advances in "keyhole surgery" in other fields encouraged surgeons also to develop a minimally invasive technique in nephrectomy. The benefits of what is known as "laparoscopic nephrectomy" include less pain, shorter hospitalisation, rapid return to normal activity, and improved cosmesis (a scar pattern of a few very small incisions, which heal almost invisibly). I shall be discussing the developments in this exciting technique in a later chapter.

Fig. 1.11 shows the pattern of incisions used for kidney removal using the method of "keyhole" surgery.

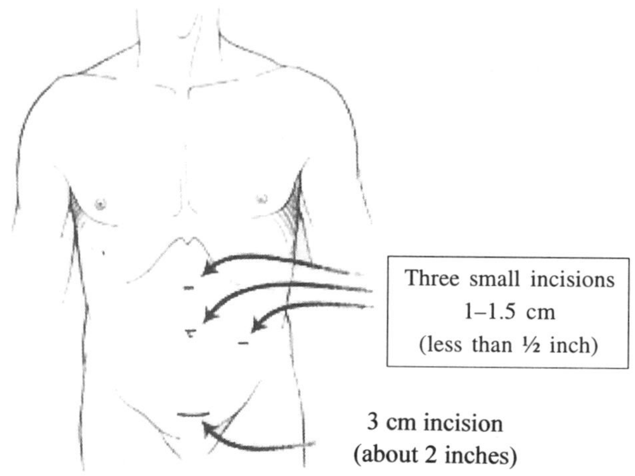

Figure 1.11   Illustration of typical operative incisions (ports) for laparoscopic donor nephrectomy. (Courtesy Johns Hopkins - Brady Urological Institute)

1.4. The Development of Microsurgery

We saw how Alexis Carrel, in 1902, demonstrated a new technique for joining the two parts of severed arteries. He continued to persevere in this extremely exacting field of vascular anastomosis (an artificial connection between two tubular organs) He also performed a number of successful autotransplants (relocation from different parts of the same person) of kidneys, toes and fingers, which required joining together very small blood vessels, and severed nerves and muscles

Later the American surgeon Harry J Buncke began trying to sew together the very small (1 mm) blood vessels in rabbits' ears. His early attempts were not entirely successful, and it was not until he began using a microscope, that he was able to carry out effective toe-to-thumb transplants on monkeys. This was made possible by the use of the delicate instruments and sutures developed in collaboration with engineers from Silicon Valley. These successes led to the founding of the Microsurgical Unit at the Davies Center in San Francisco, where hundreds of microsurgeons have been trained and thousands of human replants and transplants have been performed. Buncke, almost the father of modern microsurgery, edited a monumental book on the subject (5).

1.4.1. The Use of Microscopes

Early microsurgical operations relied on the eyesight and the steadiness of the hands of the surgeon. However, it soon became clear that some means of magnifying the image of the site was essential. In 1921, the Swedish surgeon C O Nylen used a single eyepiece microscope to operate on the small bones of the inner ear.

A further step towards greater accuracy resulted from the use of binocular microscopes, which gave the surgeon a sense of depth. The ways in which microscopes are used vary considerably: in some cases the ocular systems are worn by the surgeon like a pair of highly magnifying spectacles, while in others (Fig. 1.12) the microscope is mounted centrally and contains a number of eyepieces, so that several members of the team can look at the same time. As an additional aid, the image, or images, from one or more microscopes may be displayed on a video screen. Such a process is, of course, capable of extension so that the images can be transmitted and shown anywhere in the world.

1.4.2. The Application of Microsurgery

The Oxford Concise Medical Dictionary notes in its definition of microsurgery "....The technique enables surgery of previously inaccessible parts of the eye, inner ear, spinal cord and brain (eg for the removal of tumours and repair of cerebral aneurysms), as well as the re-attachment of amputated fingers (necessitating the suturing of minute nerves and blood vessels) and the reversal of vasectomies."

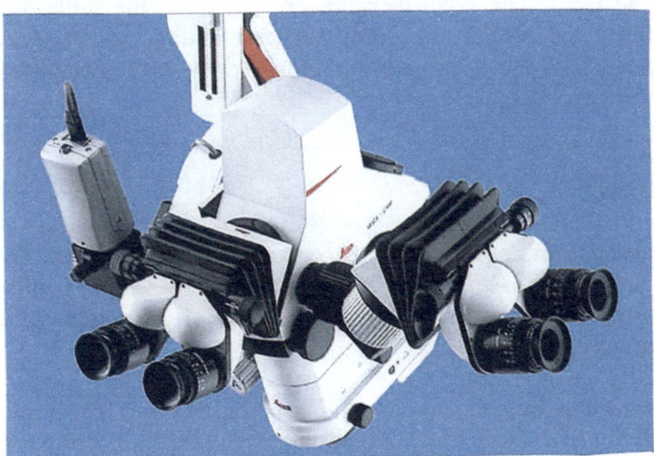

Figure 1.12 A multi-eyepiece microscope, which can be mounted on an arm above the operaing table (Courtesy Leica Microsystems (UK) Ltd)

There are other applications, of course, and we can make the general case that tiny nerve repairs and grafts are ideal for the microsurgical approach, as well as vascular repairs in and around the hands.   In summary, therefore, we can say that microsurgery is indicated for, amongst other things:

* Hand Reconstruction
* Nerve Compression and Repairing Severed Nerves
* Nerve Injuries - Repairs and Grafts
* Tendon Repairs and Reconstruction
* Skin Grafts and Flaps
* Finger Transfer
* Arterial and Venous Repairs
* Vasectomy Reversal and Male/Female Fertility Correction

It will be sufficient here, in order to illustrate the skills involved, only to deal with a couple of these categories: one of them is highly dramatic, the other rather less so.

Facial Nerve Grafting

Unilateral Facial Nerve Paralysis arises from a number of causes: newborn babies' birth trauma, tumour removal, or a condition known as "Bell's Palsy". One of the most successful methods of treatment to achieve facial symmetry, and the ability to smile, is by a microsurgical technique—Cross Facial Nerve Graft—whereby a graft from the sural nerve in one of the patient's legs is carefully dissected out and implanted in the face. The 1 cm incisions are hidden in the smile lines on either cheek. Generally the results are highly successful, although movement may be lacking in the upper eyelid. This can be improved by the implantation of a small gold weight in the eyelid.

Hand Transplantation

Whilst reconstruction of the tiny tubes that are arteries, veins, nerves and ligaments in the hands, and the replacement or transplantation of severed or missing fingers, are now almost routine, the successful replacement of a severed hand remains a comparative novelty.

A hand transplant was attempted in 1964 in Ecuador, but it was rejected due to the inadequacy of the available immunosuppressive agents. After several other partially successful attempts; finally, in 1998 in France, a team of doctors performed a hand transplant on Clint Hallam - a New Zealander. Three years later the hand was amputated in London at the patient's request. It was reported that he had not followed the recommended anti-rejection treatment and physical therapy.

The attachment of the severed hand to the stump of the arm is an exceedingly complex orperartion. It involves not only joining together the blood vessels, nerves, tendons and muscles., but may also include the attachment of metal plates or rods to provide additional support. Fig. 1.13 shows the two components prepared for joining together, and the restored hand some time after surgery.

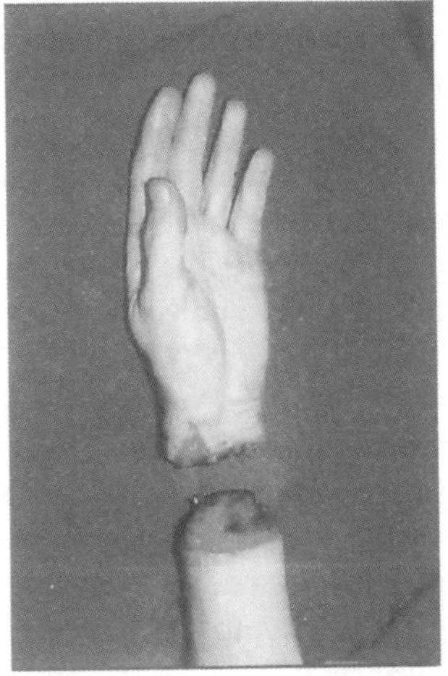
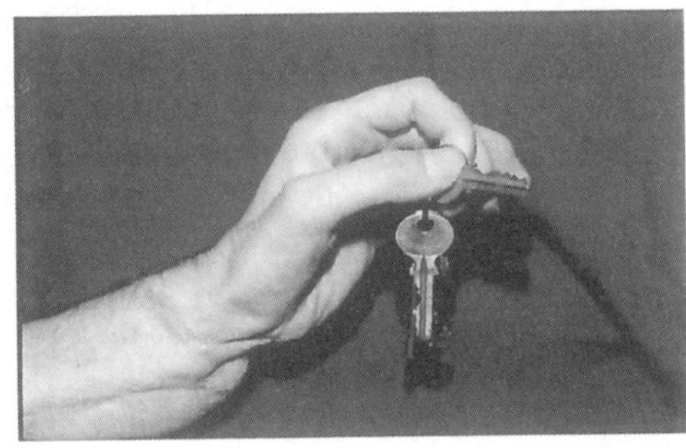

Figure 1.13 A hand ready for transplatntation onto the prepared foream, and the restored hand after surgery (Ccourtesy Mr Michael Brough, The Royal Free Hospital, London)

In 1999, and again in 2001, two patients received hand transplants at the Jewish Hospital, University of Louisville, USA, and—although it is too soon to judge the long-term outcome—both are responding well, the former gaining strength, control and a good range of motion in the new hand. The operation is extremely complex, taking from 13-17 hours, in which many very small vessels have to be trimmed and reconnected.

Double hand transplants were also performed in 2000 in Austria and France, on two patients whose hands were blown off in explosions.

1.5. Conclusion

The topics we have so far covered in this chapter represent the surgical techniques developed for operations which entail the removal and replacement of some diseased organs, and the repairs to those which are faulty or damaged. I am very conscious though, that in a profession which is able to repair, replace or remove virtually every part of the body, I have had to leave out many surgical procedures, including the treatment of varicose veins, eye surgery &c. I have also deliberately omitted to describe the highly sophisticated and intricate surgical techniques which have been carried out on children and very small babies. In the latter case, the heart is only the size of a plum! These are often modifications of those developed for, and practised upon, adults. One brief mention might be appropriate, however, the angioplasty (see Chapter 5) procedure recently carried out successfully in London to clear the blocked artery of a child, who had his first heart attack when a few weeks old, and the second aged only two years.

I hope, however, that what I have covered will be sufficient to make the reader aware of the tremendous advances that are being made across the field of surgery. This being the case, it is worth mentioning that in certain areas the rate of advance is so rapid that what is considered ground-breaking today, will tomorrow be looked upon as routine, and the sights raised once again.

It should also be remembered that the motivation for this quest for perfection owes its being to the desire, not simply to perform operations on parts of the body hitherto not amenable to surgery, but mainly to achieve these ends with less pain and trauma to the patient. Apart from the obvious benefits of reducing the mental and physical anguish, more rapid recovery is achieved, together with cost savings on reduced bed occupancy and more economical use of staff time.

As I indicated at the start of this chapter, we shall—while considering materials for specific applications—deal briefly with the surgical procedures involved in their use. These include orthopaedic surgery (involving eg the replacement of hip, knee and ankle joints, and those of the arm), artificial heart valves, as well as other types of reconstructive and cosmetic surgery.

References

(1)   Grabel J C., *Gamma Knife Radiosurgery,* Gamma Knife Center, Florida (2001)
(2)   Hoarstrup H., *American Genetics News.* Dec. 19 (1999).
(3)   Robl J., *New Frontiers in Tissue Engineering.* Innovation , Dec. 16 (1997)
(4)   Sims N. (ed), *The Heart & Circulatory System* (Reader's Digest, London 2000).
(5)   Buncke Harry J., ed, *Microsurgery:Transplantation Replantation* (Lea & Febiger 1991).

Chapter 2
Material Properties

2.1. Introduction

Synthetic materials are finding increasing applications in medicine and allied fields and, in particular, the role of plastics is becoming more important. There are also many instances where different materials, either singly or in combination, are uniquely suited to solve a particular medical problem. A typical example is the pacemaker, an implantable battery-powered device whose function is to stimulate and regulate the patient's heart rhythm under a wide range of conditions.

This, and other devices, will be considered in more detail in subsequent chapters, but it is sufficient here to understand that a modern pacemaker contains in its makeup a mix of plastics, rubbers and metals, which have to contend with two quite different sets of problems:

* Mechanical – ie robustness, fatigue-resistance. lightness
* Chemical – ie acceptable to the body and impervious to its fluids

The spectrum of materials available for use in medicine is made up of three main classes: metals, ceramics and polymers (plastics and rubbers), each with its own characteristic range of properties. In order, therefore, to be able to decide which material to use, and to derive the maximum benefit from it, it is essential that its place in the spectrum is thoroughly understood—what it can and, equally important, what it cannot do.

2.2. Structure/Property Relationships in Materials

All materials are made up from assemblies of atoms, and there are two principal factors which control the properties of the material:

* The nature and variety of the atoms (building bricks)
* The arrangement of the atoms in space (how they are put together)

The importance of both factors in determining materials' characteristics is strikingly demonstrated by considering the two neighbouring atoms in the table of elements; carbon (C) and nitrogen (N). The former is a solid at room temperature, and remains so up to $3500^{0}C$, while the latter is a gas at room temperature, and is only solid between $-210^{0}C$ and $-196^{0}C$. Also the way in which the atoms are disposed in the solid carbon accounts for the difference between the hard glossy diamond, and the grey greasy graphite. In the case of diamond, the carbon atoms are all strongly bonded together in a dense three-dimensional structure (see Fig. 2.1a).

29

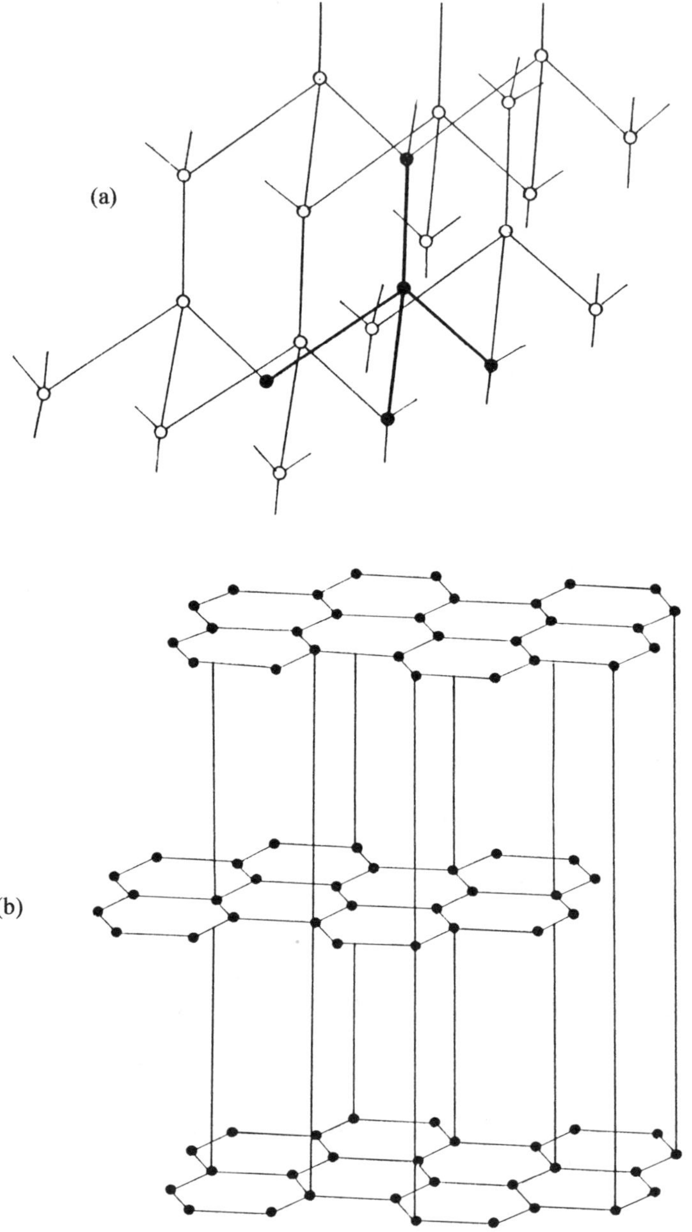

Figure 2.1 Two examples of the structure of carbon, (a) diamond (b) graphite

In graphite, the carbon atoms are arranged in sheets which, because of the relatively weak bonds between them, can slide over one another (see Fig. 2.1b)

Now that we can appreciate the importance of atomic and molecular architecture, it will be appropriate for us to consider some of the ways in which we can create different properties in the three classes of materials.

2.2.1. Metals

It is convenient to start with metals, not only because they are the most familiar of the engineering materials, but also since an appreciation of the fundamentals of their structure/property relationships will make it easier to understand the behaviour of polymers.

The majority of metals consist of relatively simple, close-packed assemblies of atoms arranged in a framework—the crystal lattice—(see Fig. 2.2). By altering the shape and structure of the crystal lattice, it is possible to generate a range of different properties.

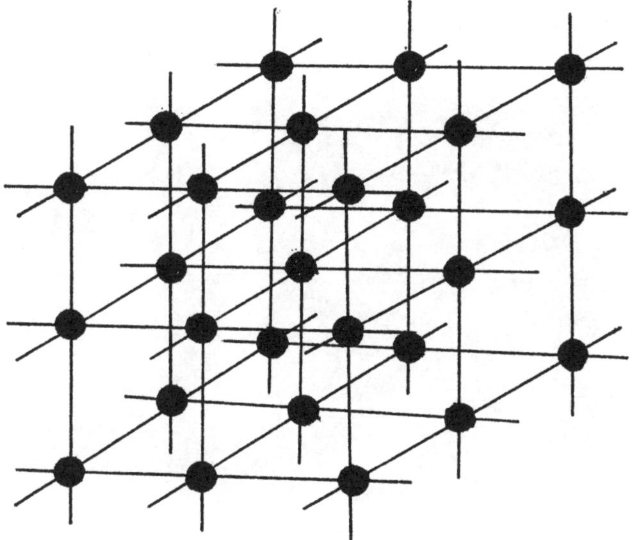

Figure 2.2 The arrangement of atoms in a crystal lattice

So far, in this brief introduction to the properties of materials, we have concentrated on so called "pure" structures where their characteristics are generated by only the type and arrangement of the constituent atoms. We must now consider what happens if we introduce an imperfection or foreign substance into the crystal lattice.

The Introduction of Imperfections into the Crystal Lattice

When pure metals are subjected to an external pressure, it is possible for the planes of atoms to "slip" past one another, and the metal deforms. The presence of a fault, or "dislocation", in the crystal structure weakens the bonds holding it together, and allows the material to slip more easily. This reduction in strength, compared with that of the pure crystal, is typically in the region of 100 orders of magnitude. We can, however, control this phenomenon by the incorporation of soluble foreign atoms which, by reducing the tendency to slip, strengthen the material. A typical example is the addition of zinc (Zn) atoms to copper (Cu), to produce brass alloys.

The Effect of Grain Structure

Engineering materials are rarely used in the form of single crystals, but normally, because of the ways in which they are manufactured, consist of a mosaic of differently oriented crystals—or grains—(see Fig. 2.3).

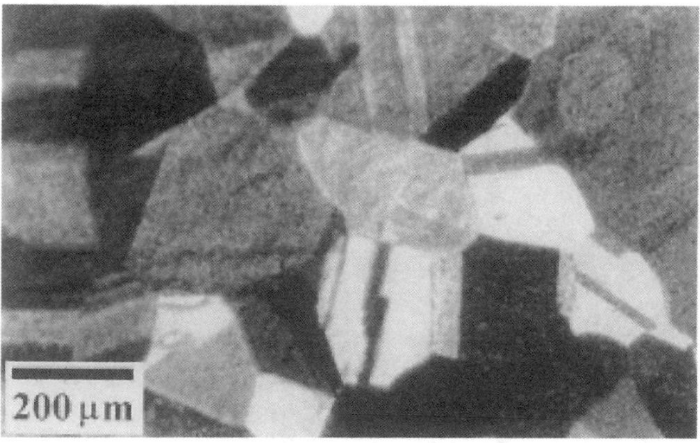

Figure 2.3 Illustration of grain structure in an austenitic steel

The size, shape, structure and orientation of the grains can be varied by mechanical working and heat treatment, and these processes will influence the physical properties of the resulting material.

The Introduction of a Second Phase

The movement of faults or dislocations under applied stress can often be inhibited by the introduction of small particles (the disperse phase) throughout the host material. The most familiar example is that of steel; which is produced by the introduction of small quantities of carbon (C) into pure iron (Fe). The use of temperature (heat treatment)—the amount by which the molten mass is heated and the rate at which it cools down—as well as mechanical working, which orients and consolidates the grain structure, both serve to control the amount and size of the carbon particles, and hence the mechanical properties of the resulting material. The nature of the dispersed atoms, for example Nickel (Ni), Chromium (Cr), Tungsten (W) or Vanadium (V), not only controls the strength of the resulting steel alloys, but affects their resistance to corrosion and reaction to body fluids; an important factor in the choice of materials for implantable medical devices in dentistry, orthopaedic and cardiac surgery. A brief survey of the effect on steel properties achieved by altering the disperse phase is shown in Table 2.1.

Table 2.1 The effect on steel properties of varying the nature of the disperse phase

Composite System			Disperse Phase - Variables Changing		
			Shape	Size	Concentration
Phase			Plate to Round to Fibre	Increasing	Increasing
Continuous	Disperse	Property			
Iron	Carbides	Toughness	Increase	Decrease	Increase
		Hardness	Decrease	Increase	Decrease

In this short description of metals and their properties, we have seen how the choice of appropriate atoms, and the control of their disposition in space, has allowed us to create a whole range of useful characteristics.

It is worth noting here that, as we shall see later, the use of many of these techniques may be applied to generate desirable properties in the other classes of materials.

2.2.2. Ceramics

Ceramic materials contain phases which are compounds of metallic and non-metallic elements. There are many ceramic phases because:

* There are many possible combinations of metallic and non-metallic atoms
* There may be several structural arrangements of each combination

Most ceramic materials, like metals and some polymers, have crystal structures; however, unlike metals—where the electrons are free to roam around the atoms forming the crystal lattice—the electrons in ceramic structures remain close to the atoms forming the skeleton of the structure. This freedom to roam, incidentally, is what allows metals to conduct heat and electricity so easily.

In the case of ceramics, the electrons which form the bonds between adjacent atoms, are either shared between them—which produces extremely strong links (known as covalent bonds)—or are transferred from one atom to another giving slightly weaker links (known as ionic bonds). The way in which this happens is shown in Fig. 2.4

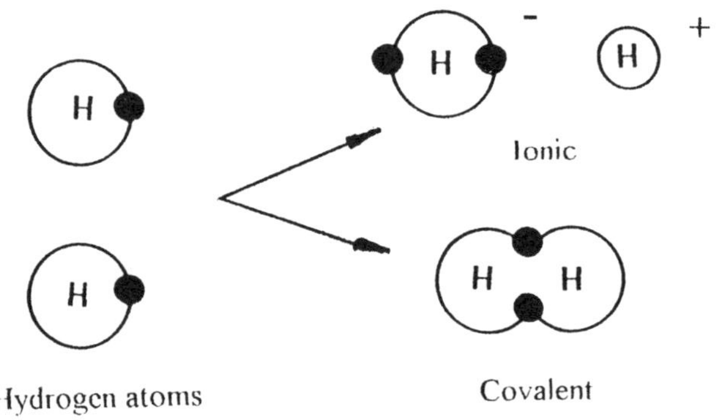

Figure 2.4 Electron transfer between hydrogen atoms to form the hydrogen molecule. In the former case an ionic bond is created; in the latter a covalent bond results.

In some of the simpler crystals, such as magnesium oxide (MgO), plastic slip—similar to metallic slip—can occur. Crystal outlines can also form during growth, as for example in the cubic outlines of the grains of common salt (NaCl).

In asbestos the crystals have a marked tendency to form long chain-like structures; while in micas and clays the crystals form two-dimensional sheet structures. The stronger, more stable, ceramic materials commonly possess three-dimensional network structures with equally strong bonding in all three directions.

The ability to choose betwen the three types of structure, and the freedom to adjust the properties of the chosen structure by the incorporation of different metallic atoms, provides us with a useful range of materials for dental applications—cements, crowns, inlays and cosmetic "veneers". There is also increasing scope for the hard-wearing and smooth-surfaced ceramics as components in orthopaedic surgery: ball and socket joints.

2.2.3. Polymers

In metals and ceramics the atom, the ion and the crystal lattice are the important features in determining properties. In the case of polymers (of which plastics are one of the members of the family), the polymer chain is the dominant feature. It is the nature of the chain links (their size and shape), together with the ways in which the links are arranged to form the chain, the length of the chains and their disposition in space, that determine the nature of the material.

In that connection there are essentially two types of plastics: thermoplastics and thermosetting plastics (thermosets). The former can, when heated, be processed and re-processed; the latter—on heating—undergo a chemical reaction and acquire a permanent "set". The simplest analogy is what happens when we boil an egg; it cannot be made to revert to its original state. Thermoplastics, too, find a parallel in nature; namely in animal horn which, from earliest times, was softened by heat and pressed into shapes, which were retained on cooling. We shall return to the concept of the dual nature of plastics later when we come to consider how we can create specific polymer properties.

The Polymer Chain

The concept of the polymer chain was first put forward in 1922 by the German chemist Hermann Staudinger (1881–1965), who was awarded the Nobel prize for chemistry in 1953. The term "polymer" for these long-chain configurations, which include rubbers as well as plastics, was derived from the Greek by combining the two words "polus" (many) and "meres" (parts). "Plastics" evolved from the Greek word "plasticos", meaning capable of being moulded or formed. Staudinger postulated that these polymer chains were formed from many thousands of simple molecules (ethylene, propylene, vinyl chloride &c.), described as "monomers" (single parts).

The simplest type of polymer, which may conveniently be described as a one-dimensional macromolecule, consists of a single chain of backbone atoms, and the most familiar member of this class is polyethylene—where the building bricks, or monomers, are molecules of ethylene gas—derived from the fractional distillation of crude oil and natural gas.

We can gain an idea of the size of the polymer chain if we appreciate that the ethylene molecule is about 2×10^{-10} metres long, and that a typical polyethylene chain of some 50,000 links would be about 10^{-5} metres in length (in the region of one hundredth of a millimetre).

The polymer chains are normally tangled and randomly coiled, like the filaments of a bundle of wire wool. Because of this configuration the material is flexible, since rotation of the chain segments can easily occur. It is also tough, because rotation will absorb sudden stresses. It is light, because there is a large space/chain ratio (often further increased by the addition of branches in the main chain structure), and it has a low softening point, because the chains can easily disentangle and slide past one another when thermal energy is supplied to the material.

Methods of Creating Specific Properties

(a) Greater Flexibility

The flexibility of the polymer molecule, and hence the material, can be increased by a variety of techniques: most simply by the addition of plasticisers and processing aids. These additives are, in simple terms, liquids which fill up some of the voids between the chains, and so make it easier for them to move about relative to one another. This technique is most frequently used in PVC (polyvinyl chloride) technology.

However, with some plasticisers there is the possibility that they may migrate, or "leach out" from the fabricated article, and the polymer manufacturers are currently evaluating a new range for medical applications. The use of mould release agents, to facilitate the removal of the fabricated article from the mould, is also not free from problems; in that recently a very large number of ceramic hip replacement components had to be recalled because the mould release chemical had been found to impair the regenerative process once the joint had been implanted. In such applications it is obviosly best not to use additives but to modify the process. Flexibility can also be increased by the technique of co-polymerisaion, whereby some of the links in the polymer chain are replaced by ones that can more easily be deformed. The different molecular units may be combined in the polymer chain in three ways: randomly, in blocks or as branches, producing a range of properties proportional to the spatial and chemical mix of the ingredients. It is also possible to generate a further mix of properties by combining several of these different variations in the same chain.

(b) Enhanced Rigidity

On the other hand we can also decrease molecular flexibility, and this is achieved by the use of two different techniques:

(1) Physical—in which the polymer chains may be made longer, and induced to lie closer together, or by stretching in order to make the molecules to line up in a desired direction. This can produce a crystalline structure similar to that in metals.

(2) Chemical—where bulky molecules may be introduced into the polymer chain, and thus inhibit rotation. We can also design rigid molecules where the segments can rotate, but the chain itself does not bend.

The process can be carried a stage further by putting in a series of struts to produce very stiff ladder-like chains that will neither rotate nor bend (examples are carbon fibre and "Kevlar"). Finally, we can join up all the chains by chemical links to form a rigid three-dimensional network (thermosets).

An interesting technique for enhancing polymer properties has been developed recently at Northwestern University in the United States (1). Professor Samuel I Stupp found that when certain molecules were dissolved in a monomer, such as styrene, they had the ability to form ribbon-like structures only a few nanometres (10^{-9} m) wide. These strands could then be made to link up to form a scaffold–like structure. During the next stage of the polymerisation process, other molecules could be induced to align themselves around the scaffold in an orderly manner; producing changes in the optical and mechanical properties of the material.

We mentioned earlier the effects obtained by incorporating liquids (plasticisers) in the polymer mix. Other forms of additives can also produce different properties. Gases give rise to foams - either rigid or flexible; while solids - when finely divided - act as fillers, extenders and pigments. When fibres—either chopped, in skeins or woven mats—are used, the resulting materials are known as "reinforced plastics", and the engineering properties are greatly enhanced. The specific directional properties will depend upon the orientation of the fibres.

                    Life-enhancing Plastics

Molecular Architecture

Let us now summarise the techniques I have so far described, and see how the resulting materials fit into the portfolio of "designer polymers". A range of polymer structures, showing increasing stiffness, is depicted in Fig.2.5, and the effects of chain lengthening and stretching are shown in Fig. 2.6.and table 2.2. A selection of condensed polymer structures, which confer increased rigidity and strength, is shown in Fig. 2.7, and their effect on the maximum service temperature is compared in Table 2.3.

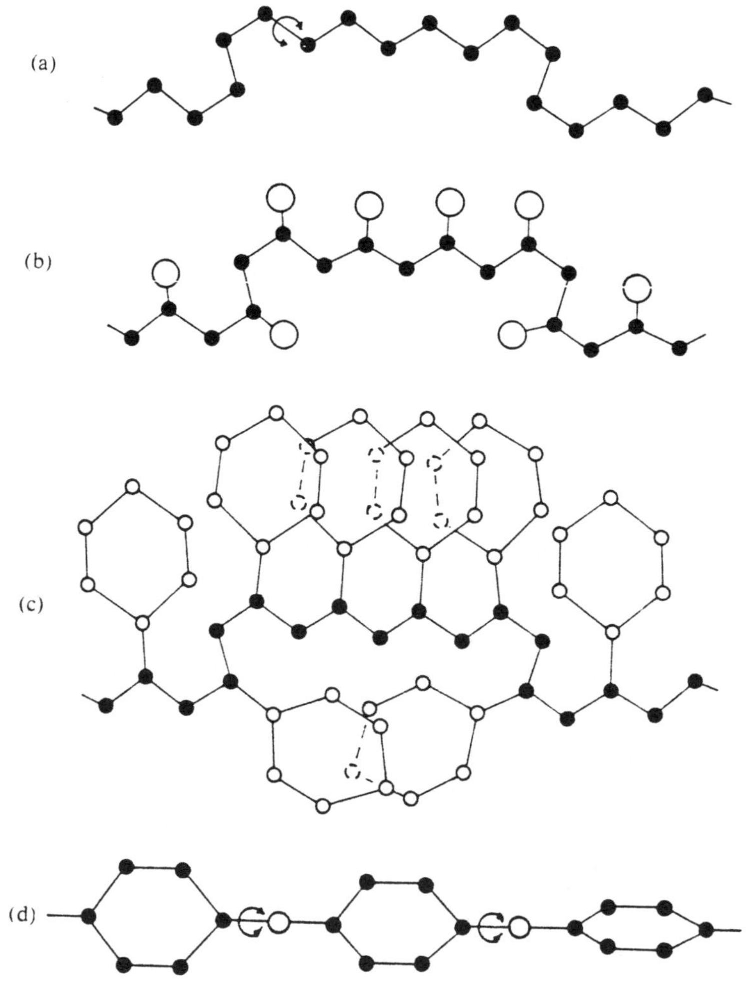

(a)

(b)

(c)

(d)

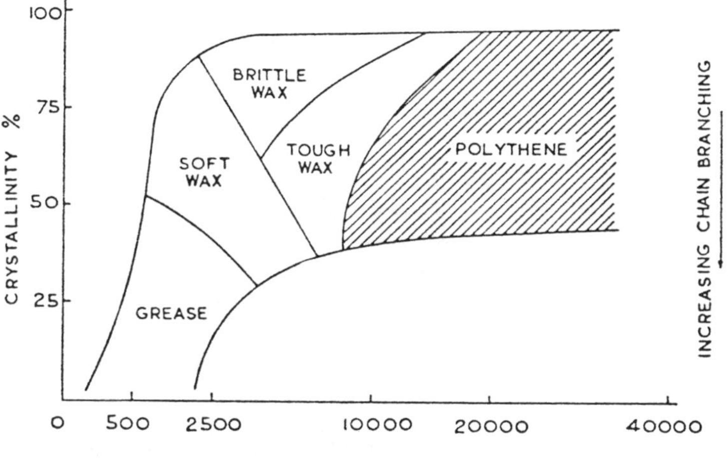

Figure 2.5 Polymer molecules of increasing chain stiffness: (a) polyethylene (b) rigid PVC (c) polystyrene (d) polyphenylene oxide (e) pilyimide

Figure 2.6 Effect of molecular weight (chain length) on polymer properties

Table 2.2 Strengths of oriented plastics films and fibres

Material	*Draw ratio*	*Stress at break* $(10^7\ Nm^{-2})$	*Type of orientation*
Polystyrene	1 : 1	3.5	Uniaxial
(film)	3.75 : 1	8.3	Uniaxial
Polyethylene	1 : 1	0.7	Uniaxial
(film)	14 : 1	13.8	Uniaxial
Polyethylene terephthalate	1 : 1	4.1	Biaxial
	2 : 1	8.2	Biaxial
("Melinex" film)	3.5 : 1	21.0	Biaxial
(fibre)	6 : 1	40.1	Biaxial
	7 : 1	55.1	Biaxial

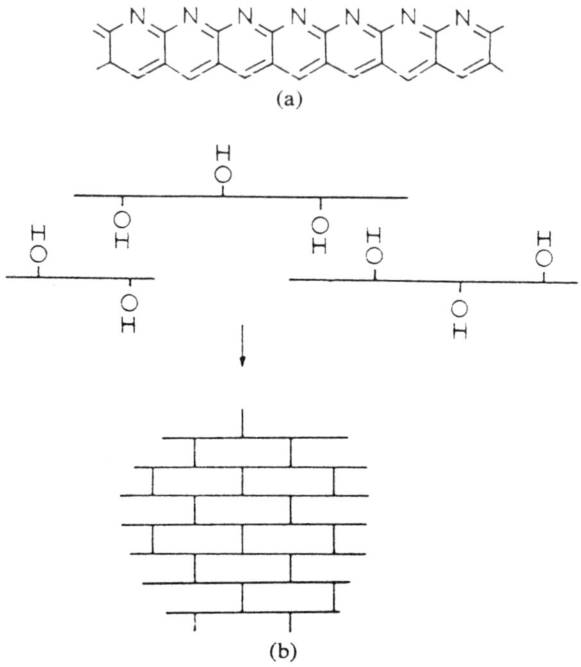

Figure 2.7 Ladder and cross-linked polymers, (a) 'Black Orlon' (b) an alkyd resin (thermoset)

Table 2.3 Maximum service temperature of plastics

Material	Chain structure	MST (^0C)
Polyethylene	Flexible	120
Polycarbonate	Rigid	135
Nylon 66	Rigid	150
Phenolic resin	Cross-linked	175
Epoxy resin	Cross-linked	235
Polyimide	Very rigid	300

Finally, we have another technique for creating specific properties: stereoisomerism. This phenomenon was originally discovered by Louis Pasteur (1822–1895) when he was working with small molecules. Stereoisomers are molecules possessing identical chemical formulae, but which have a difference in the

distribution of the atoms and chemical groups in space.   As an illustration, the
isoprene molecule (polyisoprene is a rubber) is shown in Fig. 2.8, together with its
common variants; all of which demonstrate different characteristics when formed
into polymer chains.

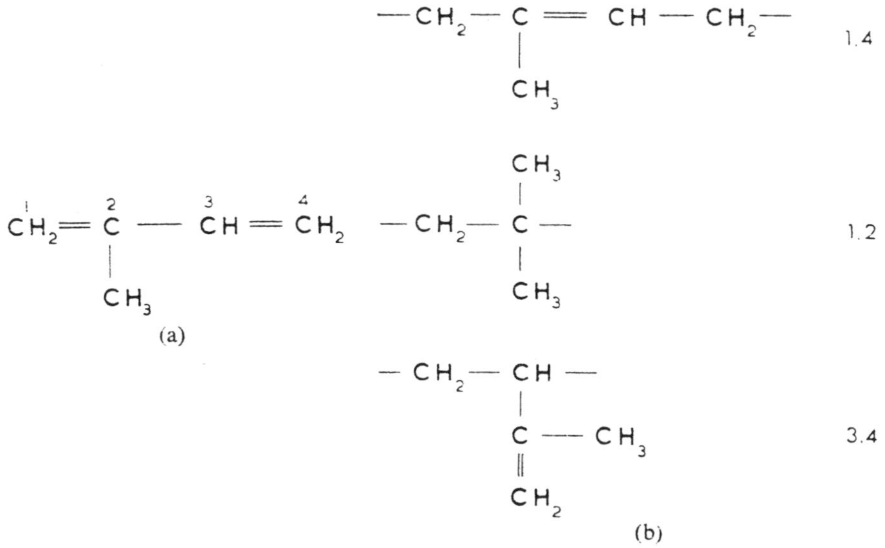

$$-CH_2-C=CH-CH_2- \qquad 1.4$$
$$\mid$$
$$CH_3$$

$$CH_3$$
$$\mid$$
$$CH_2=C-CH=CH_2 \qquad -CH_2-C- \qquad 1.2$$
$$\mid \qquad\qquad\qquad \mid$$
$$CH_3 \qquad\qquad\qquad CH_3$$

(a)

$$-CH_2-CH-$$
$$\mid$$
$$C-CH_3 \qquad 3.4$$
$$\parallel$$
$$CH_2$$

(b)

Figure 2.8 The polymerisation of isoprene, (a) the isoprene molecule (b) the different stereoisomers of
isoprene

Stereoisomers are created by using special catalysts (polymerisation inducers) which,
owing to their highly specific distribution of +ve and -ve charges, act as templates,
ensuring that the molecules can only link up in a certain way.   The use of these
special templates have found important applications in the pharmaceutical industry,
where they, in turn, are used as catalysts to ensure that   highly complex drug
molecules can be assembled in a particular way. This ensures that, when used, they
are able to reach—and lock in—to the appropriate sites in the body.

2.3. Polymers Compared with Other Materials

Having built up a picture of how polymer properties can be created, we must now
compare them with other materials, with which they might combine or compete in
service. We have to remember, however, that some of the techniques we have
considered lead to the production of very sophisticated materials, with very narrow
fields of application.

Table 2.4 provides a basic comparison between polymers and other materials, from which it can be seen that, as far as tensile strength is concerned, metals occupy about a decade centred on 10^9 Nm^{-2}. The spread for normal plastics extends from above 10^8 down to 10^7 Nm^{-2}. Foamed polymers occupy the region down to about 10^5 Nm^{-2}.

Table 2.4 Summary of the engineering properties (strength and rigidity) of materials

Material Category	Mechanical Prperties (NM^{-2})		Material Type
	Tensile Strength	Young's Modulus	
Highly condensed	10^{10}	10^{12}	Diamond
	10^9	10^{11}	Silicon carbide
Metals	5×10^9	5×10^{11}	Steel piano wire
	5×10^8	2×10^{11}	Mild steel
Reinforced plastics	5×10^8	5×10^{10}	Polyester Nylon
Unreinforced plastics	10^8	10^{10}	PVC Epoxies Acrylics
	10^7	10^8	Polypropylene
Rubbers	10^7	10^7	Elastomers
Foams	10^6		Epoxies Vinyls Phenolics
	10^5		Rubbers

We can now see that, by suitable manipulation of the types and combinations of different atoms, and their disposition in space, it is possible to design a vast range of materials; many of which are eminently suitable for medical applications. We shall be looking at a variety of these in subsequent chapters.

It is appropriate, therefore, to start with an extremely important and demanding application, where the strength and characteristics of the different classes of materials are exploited to the full. This is the field of prosthetic, or artificial, limbs; truly one where the mateials are "Life-enhancing". These devices have not only to withstand a considerable range of mechanical stresses, but also have to "look and feel right". It is right to deal with them here, since they form a bridge between the materials themselves and those applications where they come into more intimate contact with the body.

2.4. Prosthetic Limbs

In simple engineering terms, although all artificial limbs have to be strong enough to perform their specific functions as well as being able to withstand a considerable amount of wear and abuse, we can distinguish between those which have to bear the full weight of the body, the legs and feet, and those that do not, the arms and hands.

Whilst such factors as the strength, weight and resistance to corrosion and misuse of materials in prosthetic applications are important, so too is the need to duplicate, as far as possible, the tremendous range of movements and control enjoyed by the natural human limbs, as well as the sophistication of the brain, nerves and muscles which control them.

It should by now not come as any great surprise to the reader to learn that, in this field of application—as in so many other medical initiatives—pioneering work began many years ago. As the development of useful prostheses has involved some extremely ingenious uses of a wide range of materials, I thought it would be illuminating to deal briefly with the historical development of prostheses before concentrating in more detail on specific applications. One of the better expositions of the subject was provided by Northwestern University, USA, on which I have drawn from time to time (2).

2.4.1. Prosthetics from Earliest Times

The reasons for seeking the help of prostheses include: function, cosmetic appearance, and the psychological desire to appear whole. The effects and aftermath of war have also spurred the need for artificial limbs. Said to be the earliest written record of a prosthesis, the Rig-Veda (an ancient sacred Indian poem written between 3500 and 1800 BC) refers to the warrior queen Vishpla who, having lost her leg in combat, was fitted with one made of iron and returned to the battle. It was reported that the Celtic Irish god, New Hah, used a left arm prosthesis with four silver fingers.

After 500 BC we see the development of the scientific approach towards medicine and prostheses; in that the most appropriate materials then available were called into use. In Capau, Italy, a Roman prosthesis was unearthed, dating from the Samite Wars (300 BC). It comprised a wooden core, overlaid with bronze, and supported with leather straps. At about this time plays were being written (by, among others, Aristophanes and Herodotus) for actors wearing artificial limbs; a practice that was followed by an ancestor of mine—Samuel Foote, the playwright—who, having lost his leg in 1766, wrote many plays for one-legged characters; and acted in them himself!

The Dark Ages, following the fall of the Roman Empire in about 400 AD, saw a decline in prosthetic design, as such devices were generally made of iron by skilled blacksmiths, and primarily intended for use in battle. The most significant advance came with the Renaissance; in 1508, the German knight Götz lost his right arm, and ordered two iron prostheses; which were mechanical masterpieces of their time. Each joint could be moved independently by setting with the other hand, and relaxed by a release mechanism controlled by springs. The hand could pronate (turn so that the palm faced downwards) and supinate (palm upwards), and was suspended with leather straps.

In 1696 Pieter Verduyn, a Dutch surgeon, introduced the first non-locking below knee prosthesis. It used external hinges and a leather cuff, was covered with a copper shell, and had a wooden foot.

Improvements came fast, in the 1800s James Potts of London designed a leg that consisted of a wooden shank and socket, a steel knee joint and an articulated foot that was controlled by catgut tendons from the knee to the ankle.

In parallel with these developments in prostheses came improvements in amputation surgery and operating theatre hygiene (already discussed in Chapter 1). As late as 1842 Paris hospitals were reported to have mortality rates well in excess of 60%, even for the simplest amputations. It was maintained that it was safer to have a limb amputated by gunfire that by a surgeon!

The Potts leg (known both as the "Anglesey Leg", since it was used by the Marquess of Anglesey after he lost his own leg in the Battle of Waterloo, and the "Cork Leg"—because it was widely used in County Cork, Ireland)—was brought to the USA in 1839 by William Selpho, and improved in 1846 by Benjamin F Palmer, who added an interior spring, which gave it a smooth surface and concealed the tendons.

The appearance of new materials for the aviation industry enabled the British aviator Marcel Desoutter, who had lost a leg in battle, together with his engineer brother Charles, to make the first aluminium prosthesis. Later developments included pelvic (rather than shoulder) suspension, and this provided a more energy-efficient gait, greater stability and direct knee control. This, in its turn, led to further developments - such as the knee-brake (we shall understand the need for this refinement later in the chapter).

Following on the advances made after World War I, the large number of American amputees in World War II stimulated a comprehensive research program on both upper and lower body prostheses, the more significant results of which we shall discuss later.

It is evident that the artificial lambs developed over the years have attained a remarkable degree of sophistication and understanding of the use of material characteristics, and it is now appropriate to consider the two main types of prosthesis separately.

2.4.2. Artificial Legs and Feet

There are many different types of prostheses, most of which tend to concentrate on offering a particular "upgrade" over the others, so as to enable the wearer to carry out a specific task more effectively and with greater comfort. Many suppliers offer a range of leg, knee, ankle and foot components, which can be assembled in appropriate combinations to suit the particular intended activity of the wearer. Fig. 2.9 shows the components of a typical modern artificial leg. This prosthesis is a fairly simple "mechanical leg", and we shall see later how engineering skills and computer technology have contributed to making the prosthesis become more "real".

For a non-amputee the mechanics of taking a step generally go unrecognised. Therefore, before turning to the most up-to-date prostheses, it might be helpful to consider how a basic artificial leg works. In order to retain control, and avoid falling down as soon as a step is taken, quite a complex mechanism is involved. As the thigh moves forward, the knee joint is opened by inertia, the shin part of the leg moves forward, and the entire structure then locks so that the wearer can pass his or her weight over it; the knee unlocks, and the process is then repeated. The foot is sometimes rigidly attached, or uses a simple spring articulation. Using this type of system, known as "passive technology", requires far more energy to cover the same distance than that expended by non-amputees.

The goal is, of course, to devise a "smart" prosthesis, which will accommodate to different types of terrain and copy the human gait. IBM first developed such a system in 1949 and, in 1958, a Russian externally powered device was controlled from the contraction of flexor and extensor muscles. An American company, Otto Bock Orthopedic Industry Inc.—the successor to a company founded by Otto Bock in Germany after World War I—has carried the development a stage further by the introduction of the C-Leg System; the world's first completely microprocessor controlled knee/shin system, which is fitted with 'hydraulic swing and stance control'. This complex series of operations is achieved by using a PC during the fitting stage, which monitors the phase of the patient's gait, so that the knee can adapt to different circumstances. Sensors in the shin receive information from the heel and toe, as well as axial loading data, thus making it possible automatically to adjust to such changes in terrain as walking up or down a steep ramp, or negotiating stairs.

A British company, Chas. A Blatchford & Son Ltd. (trading in the US under the name of Endolite) was responsible, in the 1970s, for introducing the UK's first modular prosthetic system; which allowed a prosthesis to be assembled from a range of metal or plastic standard components, permitting combinations for most types of activity to be created. In their simplest form, these assemblies can be delivered to, and used by, the many hundreds of land-mine victims in some of the poorer countries; many of them children.   Some of these components are shown separately in Fig. 2.9.

(a)

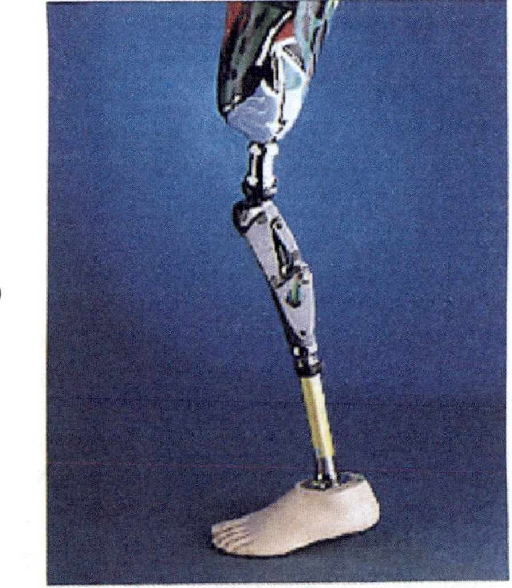

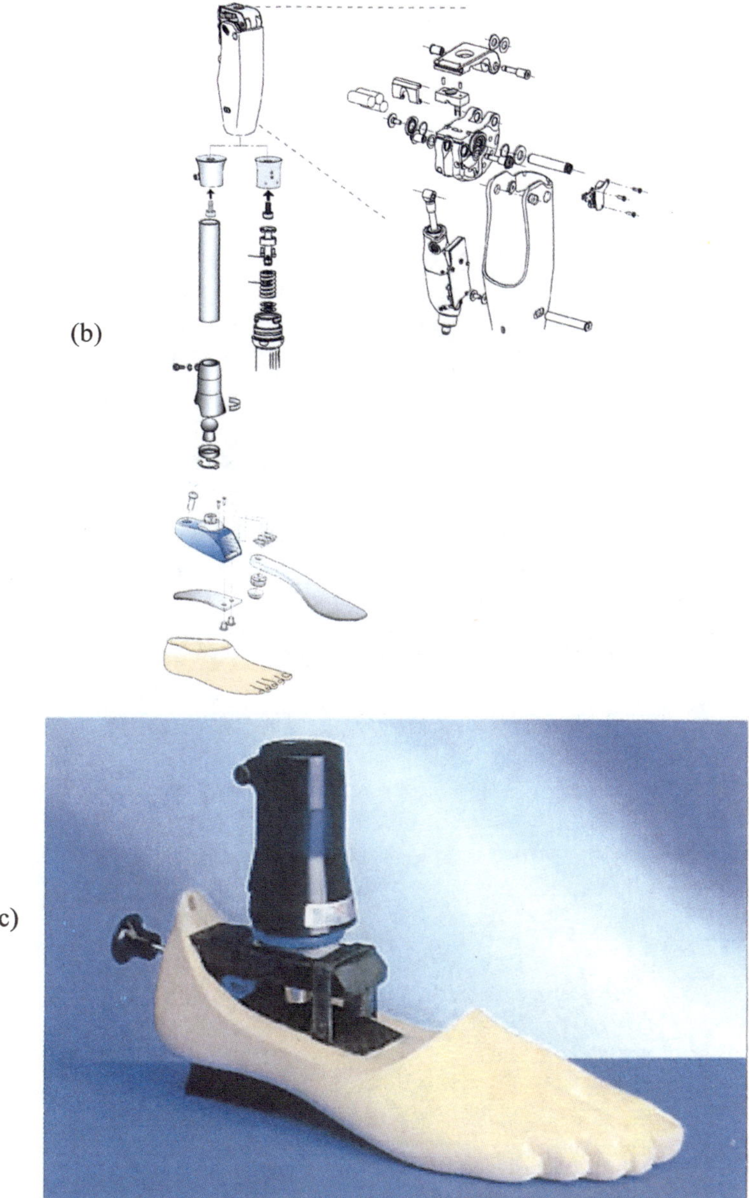

Figure 2.9 The components of a modern lower limb assembly, (a) the C-Leg systemc (Courtesy Otto Bock Orthopedic, Minneapolis, USA), (b) & (c) Separate components (Courtesy Chas. A Blatchford, Hampshire, England)

In the 1980s Blatchford produced the world's first carbon fibre prosthetic system, using materials developed for the aircraft industry. They, like Otto Bock, also offer a microprocessor-controlled prosthesis. Fig. 2.10 shows the stages in the production of carbon fibre shin prostheses.

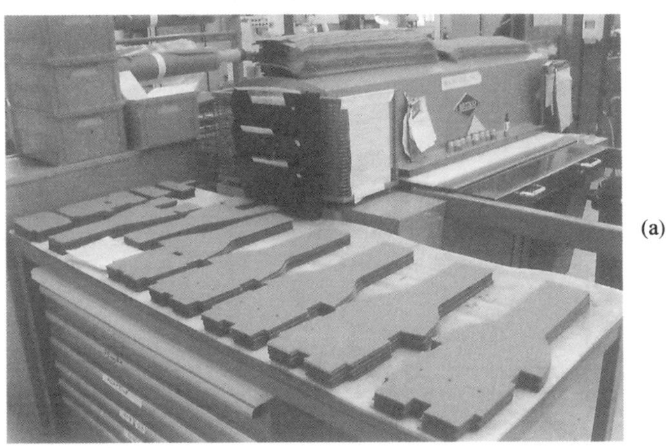

(a)

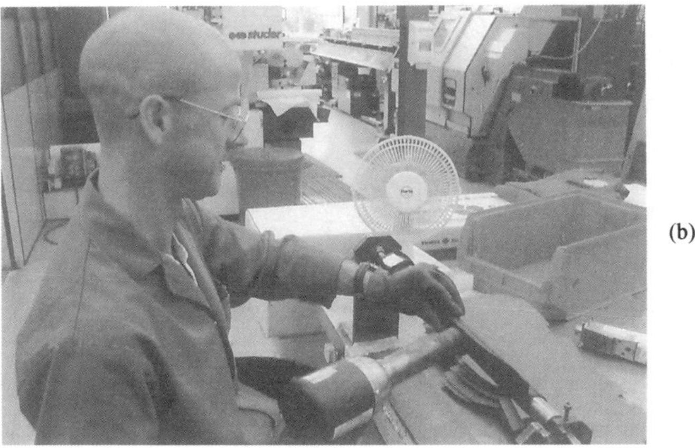

(b)

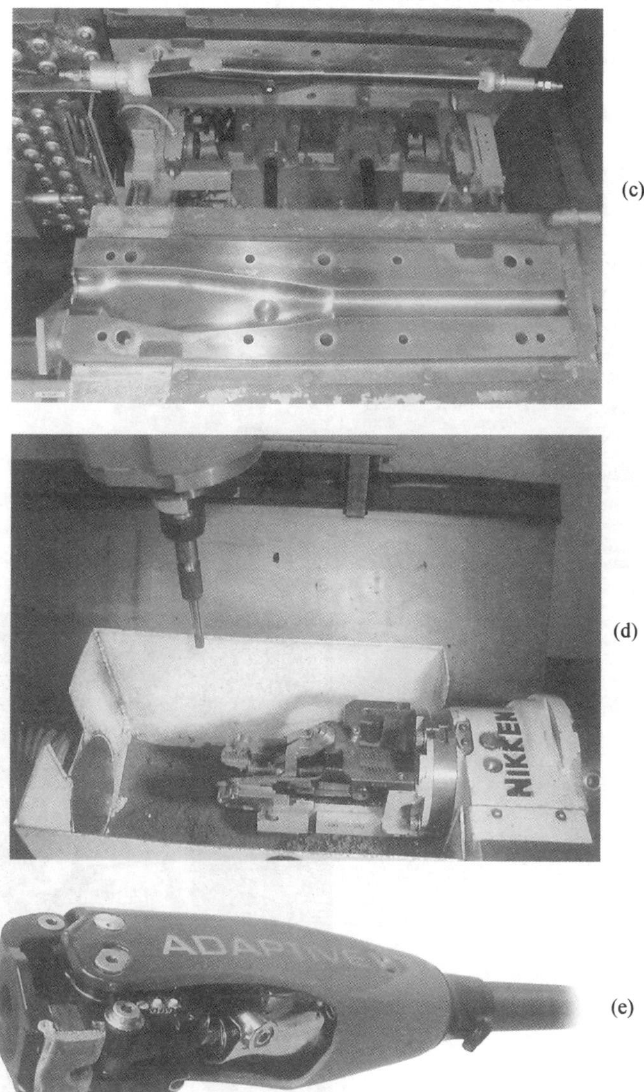

Figure 2.10 Stages in the production of carbon fibre shin components, (a) preparation of the epoxy impregnated woven carbon fibre sheets (b) the sheets are hand formed round a metal mandrel the shape of the shin, then removed and placed over an inflatable bladder (c) the preform, together with bladder, is placed in a mould, and the bladder inflated (d) the moulding is then machined to size using a computer controlled milling machine (e) the finished component. (Courtesy Chas. A Blatchford & Son Ltd, Hampshire, England)

                    Life-enhancing Plastics

Fig. 2.11 gives two examples of amputees using the modern prostheses. While not strictly necessary for high activity sports, because of the "drag", these limbs can be covered with realistic cosmeses made from silicone rubber.

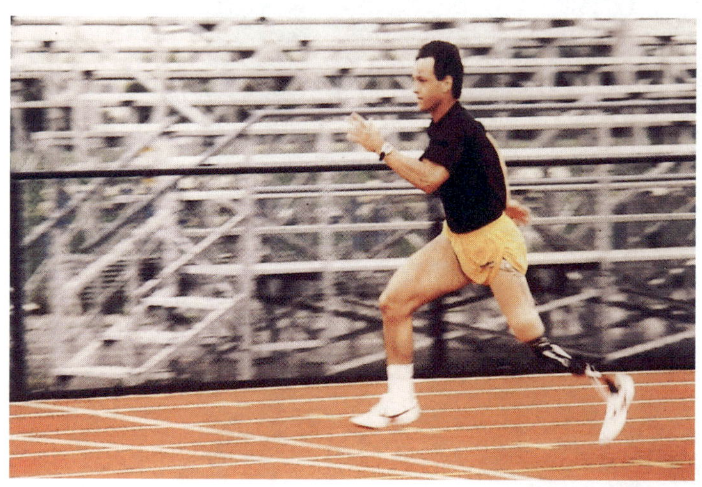

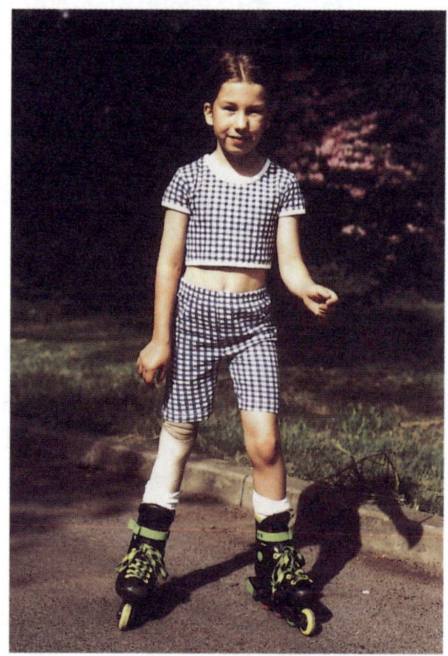

Figure 2.11 Prostheses designed for sporting activities (Courtesy Chas. A Blatchford, Hampshire, England)

It is apparent that the requirements for lower limb prostheses must be satisfied by a wide range of materials, with very differing characteristics. The ways in which they are used, together with the design of the individual components, as well as the ways in which they are fabricated, all contribute to the success, or failure, of the enterprise. Table 2.5 (at the end of the chapter) itemises mateials used in lower limb prostheses.

By way of illustratng the high degree of realism and sophistication of modern prostheses, we can consider three remarkable examples. The first is Heather Mills, journalist and model, who lost her leg in a road accident in 1993. The second is Helen Smith, who lost all four limbs in 1998 as a result of contracting meningococcal septicaemia. She was fitted with myo-electric hands (see later in this chapter) and a pair of specially constructed legs. The third is Aimée Mullins, a bilateral (both legs) amputee; who appeared on the Oprah Winfrey Show in the USA. All three are attractive and courageous women who have made no concessions to their disabilities, and by their determination have helped to show others that virtually normal lives can follow the loss of their limbs.

Materials Used in Lower Limb Prostheses

While the requirements of strength, lightness and corrosion resistance, as well as wearer comfort, are of primary importance, the outward appearance of the prosthesis contributes greatly to the self-confidence of the wearer, and much research has been carried out to develop materials which look and feel like the "real thing". Colour fastness, wear and stain resistance, together with the right degree of "spring", are matters which have taken up many years of research time. The modern silicone rubber "skins" provide highly satisfactory solutions, since moulded toes complete with toenails, can be supplied, together with realistic ankle and knee contours. It is also possible to achieve skin texture and pigmentation which matches the natural limb. Finally, developing suntan can be catered for by a series of skins with different degrees of pigmentation!

2.4.3. Artificial Arms and Hands

We have discussed the factors governing the design of an artificial leg, and the ways in which modern prostheses can be made to approximate to the human gait. However, stripped of the complexities of negotiating different types of terrain, we can see that essentially man can move forward by using the two muscle movements: flexion (bending the joint so that the bones forming it are brought towards each other) and extension (the muscular movement by which a limb is straightened); much the same as in a dog or horse. In the case of the human arm and hand the matter is not so simple.

Because humans now walk upright, the arms (forelimbs) have been able to develop a wide range of muscle movements, which make it possible to handle objects: such as tools or weapons, and to carry surprisingly heavy loads. One of the most important muscle movements that has been acquired, is the ability to oppose the thumb and fingers, using a combination of flexion and abduction (the ability to move a limb, or part of the body, away from another). Coupled with this skill is the development of dominance (left– and right-handedness), which allows a person to carry out different operations at the same time with either hand.

If we attempt to analyse the movements which can be performed by the natural arm we can divide them into several paired activities:

* Flexion and Extension
* Pronation and Supination
* Adduction (inward movement) and abduction (outward movement)

A few simple tests will show that natural movements are, in fact, almost invariably a combination of some, or all, of these simple activities.

In addition to designing a prosthesis which will perform as many of these movements as possible, in a manner which comes close to that of the natural limb, the designer has to consider how a non-amputee programs the limb to perform its chosen tasks, and how this function can be used to operate the prosthesis. An important factor, of course, is the amount of the limb which is missing; whether it is a finger, the hand, below the elbow, above it, or the whole arm from the shoulder. Also the age and size of the amputee have to be taken into account, together with the type of activity envisaged. For our purposes, however, it will be sufficient—while being aware of these additional parameters—to consider the approach to making the most appropriate artificial upper limb, and the materials involved in its construction.

The Development of Artificial Arms and Hands

We saw earlier in this chapter how, even centuries ago, prostheses were made— generally by a blacksmith—which were capable of a limited range of movements, often controlled by the other hand. Their limitations did not matter greatly, since their prime function was to enable the wearer, when mounted on a horse, to grip and hold a lance.

Little real progress was made until the turn of the 20th century, and Fig. 2.12 shows the photograph, taken in 1924, of a man wearing artificial arms. As both arms appear to have been severed below the elbow, the mechanism required for movement is comparatively simple.

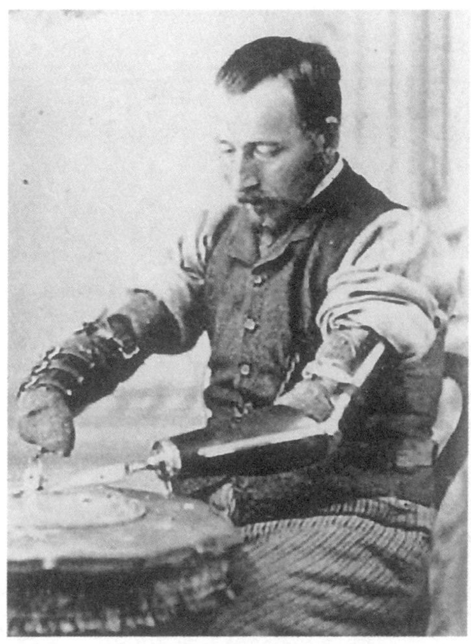

Figure 2.12 Photograph of a man wearing a pair of artificial arms (1924). (Courtesy Science Museum/Science & Society Picture Library)

The next stage in development was to provide a prosthesis that was capable of copying, at least some of the functions of a natural limb. This was achieved by a device, usually described as a "body-powered" prosthesis. In this type of prosthesis the socket fits over the residual stump, and the arm is suspended from a harness fastened around the wearer's shoulder, or upper torso. Operation of the mechanical hand, and/or elbow, is achieved by means of a cable which is activated by movements of the upper body.

Where the amputation is below the elbow, the hand—which is in the form of a hook, and works like a pair of tongs—is generally controlled by only one cable. In the case of an above elbow amputation, there are usually two cables: one flexes the elbow and operates the hand, and the second locks and unlocks the elbow joint. As with leg prostheses, the hand and arm are covered with a cosmetic outer silicone rubber skin. In the early days, plasticised PVC was used, but suffered from wear problems, and the tendency to stain and discolour. Recent advances in polymer

structure of human skin.   Fig. 2.13 shows an example of this type of mateial, which is called "Livingskin" and made from silicone polymer.

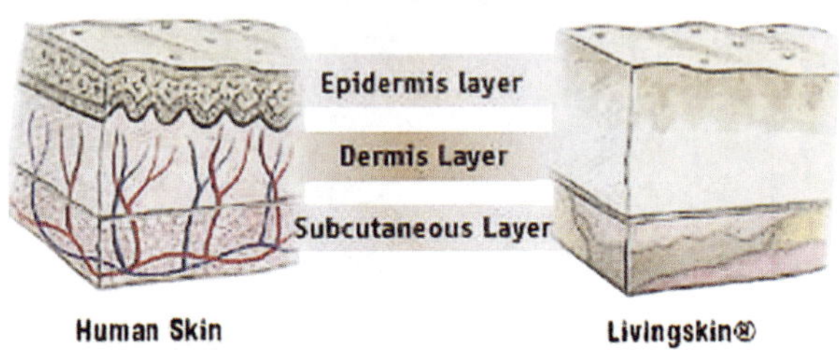

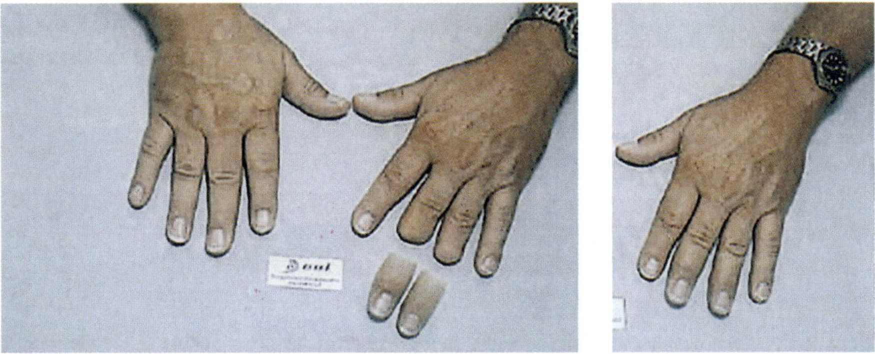

Figure 2.13 (a) A comparison of the structures of human skin and "Livingskin". .(b) examples of hand prostheses

Although the body powered prosthesis works quite well, and allows the wearer to perform many tasks, there are other limitations apart from the mechanical ones. For example, the harness tends to chafe, irritates the skin, and is difficult to clean. Psychologically, too, the harness can give a feeling of being "trussed up" and obstructed. Much research was, therefore, devoted to eliminating—or reducing—the harness, and finding an alternative to the rigid—and often painful—socket.

In the 1960s the idea of using small battery-powered electric motors to open and close the hand, rotate the wrist and flex the elbow, began to take shape. The problem was how to provide the necessary impulses to start and stop the motor. In its simplest form this was achieved in much the same way as for the cable-controlled prostheses: by movement of the limbs. Next, researchers turned their attention to nature's method: signals from the brain through the nerves, and to the muscles. At the time the brain was inaccessible and, although techniques existed for tapping individual nerve trunks they would not be suitable for everyday use. There remained the muscle; which changes both its shape and its electrical activity in response to nerve impulses. In order to use the electric current produced by muscle contraction (myo-electricity), metal discs were placed inside the socket so as to rest against the skin of the stump, and pick up myo-electric impulses. These are then amplified and used to control the electric motors which operate the prosthesis.

The pioneering work in the 1990s of an American company, Animated Prostheses Inc., led to the development of a product—known as Animated Control Systems (ACS)—to control arm prostheses (3). These are essentially a series of microcomputers, located in, or on, the arm, and pre-programmed with a power profile for each hand, so as to interpret the patient's intentions. A monitoring device, communicates with the ACS via a wireless telemetry link, so as to derive information while the wearer is using the arm. In the years followng ACS's work, a number of companies have produced myo-electric prostheses with varying degrees of complexity and sophistication. Fig. 2.14 shows an example of a modern myo-electric prosthesis.

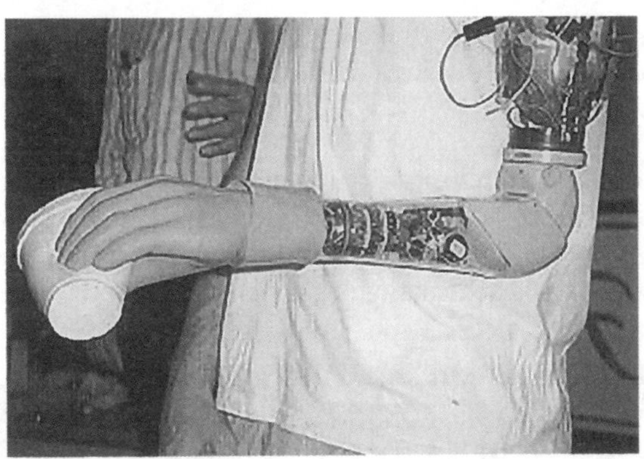

Figure 2.14 A myo-electric prosthesis

Great advances have also been made in the individual components of arm prostheses, notably in the design of wrists and hands. The Otto Bock Sensor Hand, a myoelectrically controlled prosthesis, uses small sensors located in the finger tips, together with an electronic strain gauge placed between the thumb and index finger.

The thumb is able to sense when a gripped object is about to slip. The mechanism automatically increases the gripping force until the object is again held firmly. The "flexigrip function" also allows the user to change the position of an object without causing the myo-electric control system to open and close the hand. In this way the grip appears flexible, like a natural hand.

Fig. 2.15 shows the elements of the Otto Bock Sensor Hand, together with the highly realistic silicone polymer cosmesis.

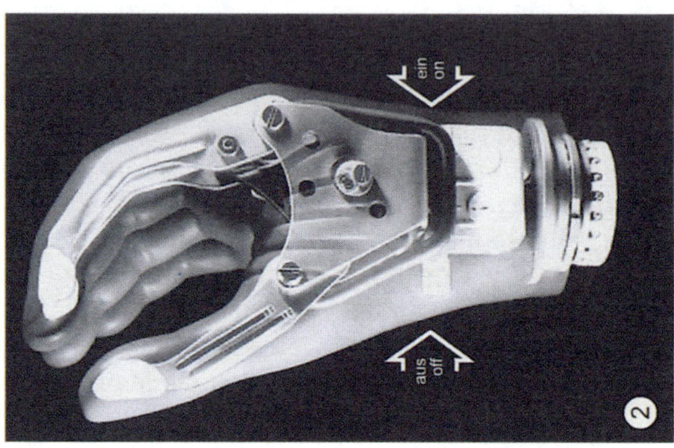

Figure 2.15 The components of the Otto Bock Sensor Hand and wrist assembly. (Courtesy Otto Bock Health Care, Minneapolis, USA)

One of the most recent examples of the application of myo-electric prostheses is that of the limbs fitted at Queen Mary's Hospital, Roehampton, Englend, to Ali Abbas, who lost both arms in the 2003 Iraq War. Fig. 2.16 gives a photograph of Ali awaiting the operation, and a achematic illustration of one of the arms.

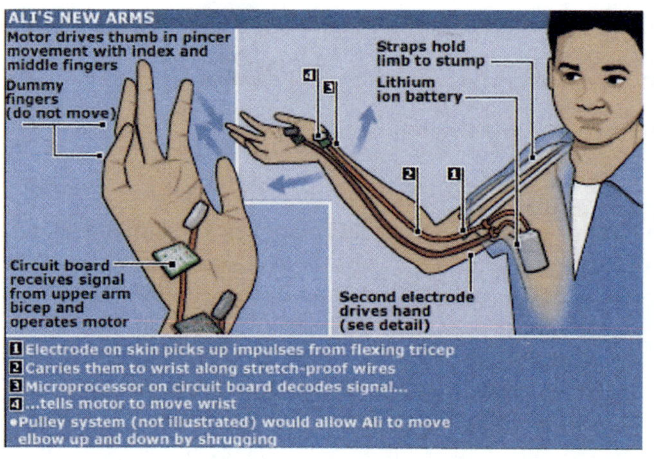

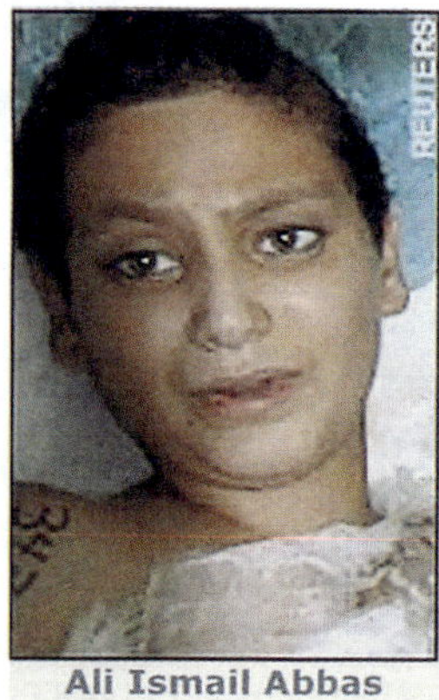

Figure 2.16 Ali Abbas and one of the artificial arms with which he has been fitted. (Courtesy The Daily Telegraph, London)

Where part of the hand and/or fingers are missing, it is possible to design and fabricate a silicone rubber prosthesis, built around an internal armature, which will not only provide the wearer with an aesthetically pleasing prosthesis, but one which is capable of gripping and holding light objects. These are, of course only partial solutions to the problem, and much research time is currently being devoted to making more sophisticated prostheses for people with parts of the hand missing or deformed. Some of these problems are mentioned below in "Current Concerns".

Current Concerns

In parallel with these developments to increase the range and quality of "natural" movements, a great deal of effort went into providing a hand that was capable of more operations than the simple hook and tong mechanism. This work has been pursued along several lines, all of them providing rewarding and exacting challenges for the engineer, medical practitioner and behavioural scientist. It will be sufficient for me to summarise them briefly here.

*   Better Mechanical Hands. The goal is to provide movement and articulation for one or more fingers, and to have a thumb that can operate separately from the other digits.

*   Sensory Perception. Currently the wearers of prostheses have to observe what happens when it is operated. Some kind of sensory feedback is needed.

*   Special Operations. Most of the current prostheses are intended for general use. Work is in progress to cater for the needs of athletes and those who perform specialist tasks.

*   Miniaturisation. Smaller limbs and components are the aim for use by children, often as young as 3 months.

*   Help for the Chair Bound. Current thinking is to make the operation of arms and hands integral with the wheelchair or other conveyance. This would also allow a longer life, and "self-charging" batteries to be used.

There are obviously other concerns for the future, including how to utilise more muscles in the operation of ever-increasingly complex prostheses, as well as the use of computer modelling to generate parts of limbs (4). Also experiments are in train, mostly with laboratory animals, to harness the brain directly in prosthetic control (5). I shall discuss these and other concepts in Chapter 8, along with other pointers to the future.

Materials for Arm and Hand Protheses

Having dealt with the range of upper limb prostheses currently available, it is convenient to consider in a little more detail the materials from which they are constructed. We mentioned at the start that, as arm prostheses do not have to bear the full weight of the body, and are rarely called upon to perform tasks requiring great strength, the materials which are used—particularly in the case of small children—should be lighter than those for lower limb prostheses. Thus we find a greater use of plastics, both reinforced and un-reinforced, aluminium and other light metal alloys, and wood. I have summarised the most common applications in Table 2.6.

In later chapters we shall deal with materials which come into more intimate contact with the body, but—before we do so—it is appropriate that we consider how to design and manufacture materials and components which are able to withstand the chemical effects of the body fluids. Equally, and perhaps even more important, we must see how to achieve components and machines which are as nearly as possible "biocompatible" with the body, and do not upset its delicate balance. This we shall do in the next chapter (Chapter 3).

References

(1) Stupp Samuel I. *Improvements in Polymers.* ACS National Meeting, San Francisco, March 30 (2001).
(2) *Prosthetics History.* Northwestern Univesity, USA
(3) *Livingskin Prosthetics Devices.* Aesthetics Concerns Prosthetics (1999)
(4) Williams N. *et al. Biomechanical Modelling and Visualisation of the Hand.* University of Sheffield. (1999).
(5) Nicolelis M. *et al.* The Brain as a Remote Control, Duke University, USA (2003)

Table 2.5 Materials used in lower limb prostheses

Application	Class of Material	Description
Support harness	Plastics	Polyester
Socket	Plastics Leather Metal	Polypropylene Aluminium alloy
Knee assembly	Plastics Metal	Polypropylene Aluminium/Steel
Shin	Plastics Metal	Carbon fibre/Epoxy Aluminium alloy
Ankle joint	Plastics Metal	Polypropylene Steel
Foot	Metal Plastics	Steel, Light alloy, Titanium Polypropylene
Small components	Metal Plastics	Steel springs & small Aluminium alloys Miscellaneous thermo- Plastic mouldings for sockets &c.
"Skin" cosmeses	Polymers	Various silicone co-polymers

Table 2.6 Materials used in upper limb prostheses

Application	Class of Material	Description
Support harness	Plastics	Polyester Nylon
Shoulder brace	Metal Polymer	Stainless steel Silicone foam
Socket	Plastics Leather Metal	Polypropylene Aluminium alloy
Elbow	Plastics Metal	Polypropylene Steel, Aluminium
Forearm	Plastics Metal Wood	Carbon fibre, Epoxy Aluminium alloy
Wrist	Metal Plastics	Steel, Light alloy Polypropylene
Hand	Metal Plastics	Titanium, Steel, Light alloy Polypropylene
Fingers	Plastics Metal	Polypropylene Steel, Light alloy
Control units (cables, motors, rods, clips & other small items)	Metal Plastics	Steel, Light alloys Polypropylene, Polyester, Epoxy
Cosmeses ("skin")	Polymers	Silicone rubber Foam

Chapter 3
Materials in a Hostile Environment

3.1. Introduction

I have deliberately used this rather emotive description of this chapter's contents since, in order to survive and continue the process of replacing and renewing dead and dying cells, the body has had to develop a method of summoning up biological forces to defeat invasion from both outside and inside itself. Therefore, although we can use a variety of substances to repair damage to—and within—the body, we have to be aware that the reaction of the body to their introduction will be a hostile one. Therefore, to use materials as effectively as possible, we have to understand the nature of the body's defense system and how it works.

3.2. The Immune Reaction

3.2.1. Early Discoveries

The study of the body's defense system (the immune reaction), began with Jenner's (1749–1823) work on smallpox in the late eighteenth century. Almost a hundred years later, it was discovered that the blood serum of animals that had been vaccinated (immunised) contained substances called "antibodies"; proteins (immunoglobulins) which attach themselves to foreign invaders, for example viral proteins (antigens), and are a vital component of the body's defense mechanism.

When the invading antigens appear, they are attacked by waves of antibodies, which combine with the antigens to neutralise them. The remaining white cells subsequently mature into cells called "macrophages", which embody the memory of the particular antigen, and become "hypersensitized". Should another invasion by the same species of antigen take place at a later date, these hypersensitized macrophages have the resources to manufacture very large numbers of the necessary antibodies with which to repel the invaders.

This explains why the first time we catch an infectious disease we show many of the unpleasant symptoms mentioned earlier, and why subsequent exposures to the same infection are usually without risk. We "catch" such diseases every time we are exposed to them; but after the first bout we are always prepared This readiness is called immunity

As our understanding of the body's response to the presence of hostile substances increased, it became evident that the mechanism was extremely complex, and that—certainly for the purposes of this book—it would only be possible to give a very simplistic outline.

The body's immunological response to invasion is known as the "immune reaction", and its mechanism—following the discovery in the 1960s that antibodies were generated by certain white blood cells called "lymphocytes"—is described clearly and readably by Donald Longmore in his book "Spare Part Surgery" (1). Part of what he says goes as follows:

> "The body's inner defense mechanisms are not concerned with any philosophical contrast like "living or dead", "friendly or antagonistic". Their activity is triggered by one single event: the appearance in the body of a chemical entity that the body can recognise as *not-itself*. That entity may be living (such as a bacterial cell) or non-living (such as the toxic chemicals secreted by a bacterial cell); it may be "friendly" (such as skin deliberately transplanted from another body to cover a wound) or "antagonistic" (such as the dust and dirt that may fall on an uncovered wound); in all such cases the body's defenses act as if they asked one simple question of these immigrant tissues, cells or chemicals: "Do I recognise this substance as self?" If the answer is "No", they set about fighting the invader.

> The gross symptoms of this fight—fever, swelling, irritation, blisters, boils, rashes, vomiting, diarrhea and so on—stress how violently the body strives to maintain its integrity, its selfhood. The fight is to the death, either of the body or of the invader. Only very rarely does the defense system withdraw its forces and, so to speak, learn to tolerate the foreign tissues. In passing, I must stress that everything I say here about the body rejecting a graft applies, mutatis mutandis, to the graft rejecting the body; after all when we put a large organ from one animal into the body of another, we are putting two immunologically mature systems against each other.

> The defense system itself centers around the scavenging white cells or *lymphocytes* that circulate like free-living organisms in the bloodstream. Like free-living organisms they are motile (capable of movement) and can engulf and digest small particles and whole cells of invading organisms."

As Longmore points out later in his book, nerve-rich tissues such as eyes and voluntary muscles do not undergo immunological rejection since they do not come into direct contact with the blood. It is for this reason that corneal allografts in the eye can be successfully performed. This behaviour is also discussed in Chapter 10.

3.2.2. Some Questions and Answers

What we have just discussed is all right as far as it goes, but—in the light of recent discoveries—a number of important questions need to be answered:

* Are there different types of lymphocytes
* Where do they come from
* How do they work
* How does the immune system distinguish between "self" and "nonself"

The Nature of Lymphocytes

Although some stem cells can produce lymphocytes, and other white cells (phagocytes) can overcome certain antigens, lymphocytes predominate in the bone marrow. One type of white cell, the B lymphocyte, continues to reside in the bone marrow until it is capable of carrying out the activities of the immune system; while the other type, the T lymphocyte, migrates to the thymus—an organ which lies behind the breastbone—where it undergoes further processing before emerging into the bloodstream.

While both B and T cells are able to attack invaders, they operate in different ways, and—for our purposes—the following simplified description will suffice. Each B cell generates specific antibodies, which are capable of recognising and interacting with specific antigens, such as bacteria and other toxic molecules, but are incapable of entering living cells where certain invaders can hide.

T cells, on the other hand, operate in two principal ways: in one, "Regulatory" T cells help the B cells to carry out their tasks. In the other, Cytotoxic T cells; killer cells as their name suggests, not only seek out and destroy cells which have been infected by viruses, or transformed by cancer, but are also responsible for the rejection of tissue and organ grafts by interacting directly with cells that have been taken over by hostile invaders.

How do Lymphocytes distinguish between "Self" and "Nonself"?

Virtually all cells carry a "marker" which allows them to be identified as self or nonself. Since the immune system has to be able to recognise many thousands of different cells, the process is highly complex. However, in simple terms, we can say that the markers which identify the cell as self are provided by a group of genes contained in one of the cell's chromosomes. These markers can be recognised by B and T lymphocytes, which themselves contain a wide variety of markers.

The recognition process is rather like a lock and key: certain combinations recognise cells as self and therefore to be tolerated. With others, the interlocking is recognised as nonself, and the appropriate destruction mechanism comes into play. Sometimes tolerance breaks down, and the T cells can generate proteins which are

                          Life-enhancing Plastics

hostile to the body, producing inflammation and possible tissue damage. This phenomenon, known as "autoimmunity", can lead to a number of serious conditions, the most common of which is rheumatoid arthritis.

A better understanding of the mechanisms involved in the immune reaction is the goal of immunological research, and the indications are that this could provide exciting solutions to many of the problems which currently exist. For example, the design of processes which selectively augment or diminish the immune response towards particular antigens would allow autoimmune diseases and other rejection mechanisms to be treated by controlling the immune response to self antigens without sacrificing the reaction to hostile pathogens. A possible treatment of cancer could lie in the generation of an immune reaction against the cancer by vaccination with the patients own cancer cells. Normally this type of reaction does not occur, since cancer cells are recognised as self and are, therefore—at least for the time being—not attacked..

3.3. Dealing With the Immune Reaction

We can now see that any intrusion into the normally peaceful functioning of the body is likely to cause a strong adverse reaction. Unfortunately, almost all the surgical procedures we have discussed involving repair or replacement, including organ transplantation, involve the introduction of "foreign" materials, either natural or synthetic, into the bloodstream.

Our task, therefore, is to plan how to cope with the immune reaction, and to make it less antagonistic to attack. In order to do this, we need to know more about blood, and in particular the following:

* The composition of the blood
* How it can be damaged
* How it seeks to respond to such damage

3.3.1. The Composition of Human Blood and its Circulation

In simple terms, blood is a tissue containing living cells, with specific functions to perform. The most important is to convey materials from one part of the body to another, so as to promote growth, repair and replacement, and the elimination of waste products. In order to do this, each living cell carries within itself all the chemical processes necessary for it to continue to exist. Therefore, all the materials which it requires must be conveyed to it, and those which it discards must be removed.

In humans, as in all higher animals, the blood consists of two major groups of components:

* The Plasma
* The Corpuscles – Red blood cells (erythrocytes)—transporters of O_2 & CO_2
                    – White blood cells (leukocytes)—defenders against attack
                    – Platelets (thrombocytes)—blood clotting agents

Although the plasma has an important function as a carrier of the corpuscles and soluble chemicals, including proteins, salts and hormones; it is the nature and role of the corpuscles which concern us here, together with how they react to adverse circumstances.

The circulation of the blood is accomplished by means of a series of smooth elastic contractions, which operate with extreme delicacy. Also, although the output of the heart takes the form of intermittent pulses, this is transformed into a wavelike, virtually continuous movement, which is also smooth and completely without turbulence.

3.3.2. The Causes of Blood Damage

Apart from events unrelated to the medical device, damage to the blood may be caused by a variety of circumstances, which fall into two main categories:

* Mechanical – the effect of pressure, turbulence, surface characteristics
* Chemical – the chemical nature of the invading surface

<u>Mechanical</u> The design of suitable pumps to circulate the blood is important. Early studies showed that blood damage due to turbulence occurred with "elastic" pumps, where sacs are sucked and squeezed alternately. The same could be said of piston pumps and centrifugal pumps, although work in the space industry has improved the performance of the latter, so that at relatively high speeds (1200–1400 rpm) they behave satisfactorily. Roller pumps and Archimedian screw devices have also been evaluated with some success, but more needs to be done.

In addition to the importance of the geometry of the blood circuitry, flow-speed is another vital consideration. For example, with replacement heart valves, more clotting problems occur with the mitral valve than with aortic valve replacements. Typically, the mitral valve has twice the area of the aortic valve, and—for approximately the same volume of blood delivered per heartbeat—remains open for twice as long. The blood flow through the mitral valve is thus slower than through the aortic valve, and we can infer that slow-moving blood is more prone to clotting.

Also, where clotting has been observed, with replacement valves, it has often been found to form in "backwaters", where it is not washed away from the component. This indicates that good flow paths, which are central to the avoidance of turbulence, are as important as material characteristics.

<u>Chemical</u>   We know that the single layer of molecules which lines the heart (the endothelium), as well as the surfaces of the major blood and lymphatic vessels, is negatively charged. We also know that the clotting mechanism may be inhibited by a number of chemical substances, the most familiar being heparin, warfarin, sulphated polysaccharides and salts such as sodium citrate (used to keep blood suitable for transfusion). All of these substances possess a high –ve charge, which appears to depress the ability of activator substances, like calcium salts, to encourage the clotting mechanism.

3.3.3. The Blood Clotting Mechanism

In simple terms the start of the blood clotting process begins with damage to the endothelium, and the connective tissue is exposed to the blood. Platelets then adhere to the collagen fibres in the connective tissue, and release a substance which causes nearby platelets to become sticky and form a plug, which provides temporary protection against loss of blood.

Whilst agglutination (discussed in Chapter 1) is a relatively simple process of antigen/antibody reaction, the clotting mechanism is far more complex. In common with much of the immune reaction, the chemical processes involved in the blood clotting sequence comprise a series of cascade reactions, each stage in the process amplifying the previous one. In the clotting process the reactions involve a number of proteins and proteases (enzymes which help to split the protein molecules).

The process by which blood is converted from a liquid to a solid state, may be initiated by contact with a foreign surface (the intrinsic pathway), or with damaged tissue (the extrinsic pathway). Both pathways converge, and the final common pathway—the reaction leading to clotting—follows the route which I have shown diagrammatically in Fig. 3.1.

When the presence of a foreign invader is detected, two of the molecules already present in the blood (thromboplastin) and a calcium rich salt (the activator), react with a third component, the relatively inactive "prothrombin". The effect of this chemical reaction is to produce the enzyme "thrombin". The enzyme then reacts upon the soluble blood protein "fibrinogen", converting it into molecules of the insoluble protein "fibrin". The fibrin molecules then coalesce into long chain fibrin polymers, forming a spongy, elastic, three-dimensional network, which surrounds the nearby red cells.

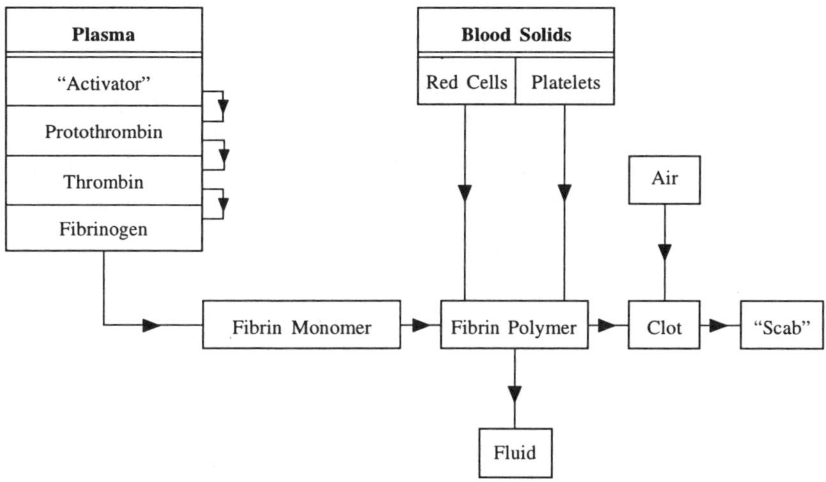

Figure 3.1 Final stages in the blood clotting process

This spongy mass receives energy from the platelets in the plasma, which causes it to contract into a firm resilient mass, and in so doing it squeezes out the plasma from the centre. Exposure to the air causes this mass to harden to form the familiar "scab" which seals a cut. Once clots begin to form they can restrict the bloodflow, and the clot (thrombus), or part of it, can become detached, and becomes what is known as an "embolus". If the embolus occurs in a vein, it can travel through the circulatory system, and become lodged in the pulmonary arteries; shutting off the blood supply to the lungs. A blood clot in an artery leading to the brain can also restrict the blood supply to the brain, sometimes with fatal consequences. We shall now have a look at some of the methods used to prevent such occurrences happening.

3.4. Designing for Biocompatibility

3.4.1. How the Scene has Changed

To begin with, biocompatibility simply meant "not interfering with the operation of biological systems". However, with the advent of more sophisticated devices, made from materials that were more responsive to local biological conditions, the principle of biocompatibility came to be regarded as "the ability of a material to perform with an appropriate response in a specific application." In particular, the design approach to implantable devices—especially long-term implants—has moved away from attempts to develop inert biomaterials, in favour of those that interact with the biological environment, and, in time, may be integrated into it. This approach is amply demonstrated by the techniques used in dentistry and jaw reconstruction (Chapter 7), and in orthopaedic surgery (Chapter 8). In the former, titanium, and titanium alloys are now widely used, and successful integration with the bone of the jaw is promoted by specially profiled surfaces, plasma spraying, or the application of a thin layer of the ceramic hydroxyapatite.

In orthopaedic surgery, too, the promotion of bone growth between the implant and the inside wall of the bone socket has been greatly enhanced by the use of a hydroxyapatite coating. Also, one of the most biocompatible metals, tantalum (Ta), has proved effective in this regard. However, tantalum is extremely difficult to transform into useful articles, and it was not until comparatively recently that a technique was devised whereby a porous, cage-like, structure in the form of the desired implant, could be made. This matrix, when implanted in the body, allows the bone-forming cells (osteoblasts) to develop and generate new bone growth throughout the preform. This process results in the formation of a strong, integrated bone/metal structure, well able to stand up to the stresses of everyday use without coming loose in the socket (2).

The materials we have so far discussed have been either metals or ceramics; and the applications are usually those in which considerable mechanical strength is required. However, there are many medical devices—such as catheters, drain tubes, angioplasty devices, and extracorporeal machines—where a flexible biocompatible surface may be needed, and this is best achieved by chemical means.

3.4.2. Chemistry to the Rescue

Ideally, what is required is a material with intrinsic biocompatible characteristics, which can be processed and fabricated into medical devices without losing these properties. Such a material is not currently available, since each application carries its own special requirements. However, it is probably not too far away.

3.4.3. Copying Nature

In the 1980s it was discovered that polymers such as polyurethane possessed an acceptable biocompatibility for many applications. However, clot formation was still a problem, and several ideas were advanced to improve the situation. These depended on the incorporation of special polymer molecules into the polymer matrix so as to form copolymers (see Chapter 2) with specific biocompatible properties.

During the last 10 years or so a number of polymer systems have evolved, and among the most successful are those developed by BioInteractions Ltd—a British company of which I am Chairman. The coating (Trillium™ Biopassive Surface developed for a series of blood oxygenators, produced by Medtronic Inc.,of Minneapolis, USA), received the Queen's Award for Innovation in 2002. The structure is shown diagrammatically in Fig. 3.2.

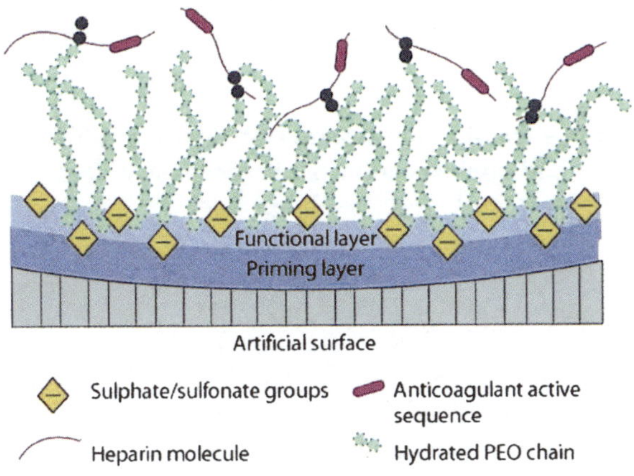

Figure 3.2 Illustration of the triple-endothelial components of Trillium™ Biopassive Surface coating (Courtesy Medtronic Inc., Minneapolis, USA)

The basic technology was developed in 1991, when Drs A K Luthra and S S Sandhu first recognised that living tissue is a dynamic system, and constantly changing. Their aim, therefore, was to create a similar mobile system, using long flexible chains—such as polyethylene oxide—on the surface of the device, so as to reduce the absorption of blood components.

During this period work was concentrated on two main polymer systems: "nonthrombogenic" and "antithrombogenic" (3) The former acts early in the clotting pathway, and prevents or reduces protein adsorption, while the latter uses materials which play an active role in preventing the clotting process. How these materials are made, and why they perform as they do, has been described in a recent paper by my colleagues Luthra and Sandhu (4),

More recently, it has been possible to combine these two characteristicss, and a haemocompatible polymer was developed with both nonthrombogenic and antithrombogenic on the same polymer backbone which provides an endothelial-like action that prevents protein adsorption and inhibits thrombin at the same time. This material (Trillium™ Biopassive Surface) works through three components: heparin, a strong negative charge and the hydrophilic (water attractive) nature of the polyethylene oxide chains.

A further development has made possible the incorporation of anti-microbial and lubricious ("slipperiness") characteristics. The former is useful in preventing catheter-related infections, and the latter facilitates the insertion of catheters and angioplasty devices (5).

I have dwelt a some length on this particular family of polymers, because they illustrate the elegance and sophistication of the chemistry used in the creation of biocompatible properties.

3.5. Conclusion

In this short chapter I have endeavoured to describe, in simple terms, the complex mechanism of the immune reaction, the response of the blood to damage, and some of the ways in which this reaction can be minimised.   An understanding of these principles will enable the reader to appreciate the size of the problem resulting from the various uses of materials in contact with body tissue, a number of which are described in the subsequent chapters.

References

(1) Longmore D, *Spare Part Surgery,* Aldus Books, London (1968)
(2) Chan S P et al, *The Osseous Response to a New Tantalum Biomaterial,* SIROT Conference, April 16-19 (1999)
(3) Luthra A K & Sandhu S S, US Patent 6,096,798 (2000)
(4) Luthra A K & Sandhu S S, *Medical Device Technology,* Oct. pp 10-16 (2002)
(5) Luthra A K & Sandhu S S, European Patent 96935033.9 (2002)

Chapter 4

Contact Applications

4.1. Introduction

It is rather unusual to start a chapter by listing the topics one is not going to include. However, it is evident that, within the definition of "Contact Applications", there are numerous devices which may come into contact with the body, but do so for such a short time that we can safely ignore them. Many of these items are disposable, and are made from plastic materials, and include for example: bedpans, urine bottles, specimen containers, plates, glasses and cutlery, wrappings and gloves. It is interesting to note in the last instance, that many hospitals and surgeries—certainly in the United Kingdom—no longer use latex gloves, since they are alleged to cause asthma in some patients. There is also the tremendous range of medical devices, diagnostic kits, machines and their attachments which are essential to modern medicine.

Now to what I shall include. In this chapter, so as to follow a logical sequence, we must consider the range of medical applications where the material in question is simply applied to the surface of parts of the body to achieve a specific function.

These include: supports (eg splints and plaster casts), dressings, contact lenses and hearing aids. The list is extensive, but—as many of the materials are similar, and can be used for a many different applications—I propose to deal only with a selection of the most typical.

In simple contact applications of this type, the hope is that, provided the device or appliance is correctly designed and fitted, the material from which it is made should not provoke any adverse reaction. However, as we shall see later, there are instances—particularly in the case of contact lenses—where the nature of the material can cause irritation, and even more extensive damage. There are also instances where the adhesive on wound dressings has caused an allergic reaction.

Let us now deal with the subject in what I hope will be accepted as a logical progression: from simple to more complex.

4.2. Dressings

4.2.1. Simple Coverings

One of the simplest applications is the use of a sterile pad to cover a wound, either freshly made, or which has been repaired by sutures or other closure devices. The pad may be of natural or synthetic fibres, and occasionally is impregnated with an antiseptic. Depending on the severity of the wound, and whether or not it needs to be kept dry, several options are available for holding the pad in place. These include bandages—again, either natural or synthetic; elastic or not—strips of woven textile or flexible plastic film backed with an adhesive. The materials used include: polyurethane (either foamed or otherwise), viscose, hydrogels and silicone elastomers, the latter frequently simply laid on the wound without adhesive, to avoid painful removal for wounds which need to be inspected frequently   Other forms of simple dressing include the "paint-on" types, which comprise a flexible plastic coating dissolved in a suitable solvent. The solution is applied with a brush or spray, and solidifies when the solvent evaporates.

4.2.2. Interactive Dressings

Where the wounds continue to bleed or "weep", as for example in the case of ulcers or burns, there is a whole range of technology available. An example—Flexipore (now sold as Spyroflex)—with which I was concerned in the 1980s, consists of a thin microporous polyurethane membrane, whose outer surface is composed of "closed" cells, and so impervious to liquids and bacteria, but highly permeable to moisture vapour and gases. The inner layer contains large voids, which can absorb and retain the exudate. The dressing is coated with a biodegradable adhesive, which allows the whole dressing to be removed safely, and painlessly, after a few days. The structure is shown in Fig. 4.1.

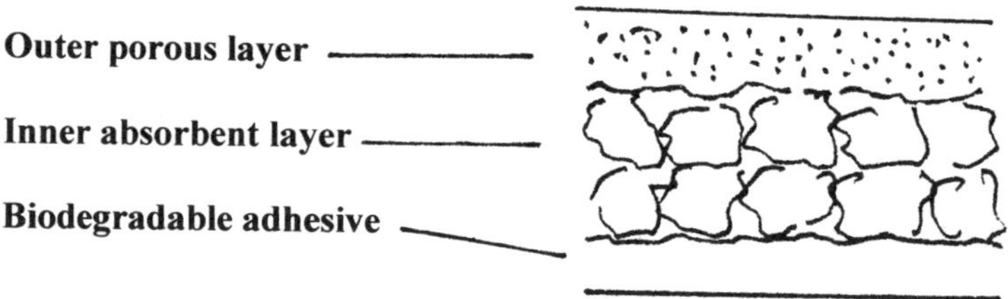

Figure 4.1 Profile of an interactive wound dressing

For some time it has been recognised that silver is a safe and effective broad spectrum anti-microbial agent for the control of infection. Indeed, in ancient times silver coins were apparently used to keep drinking water pure. One of the leaders in the field of wound care, Advanced Medical Solutions Group plc, has developed a novel wound dressing, which uses "silver fibres" (marketed under the trade name X-STATIC). These fibres comprise a layer of pure silver bonded to the surface of a textile fibre, which enables it to be incorporated into an alginate dressing, allowing a controlled and sustained release of silver into the wound.

4.2.3. Artificial Skin

There are two main types of wound which are difficult to heal:

* Chronic Wounds
* Burns

Some of the treatment procedures are similar, particularly in the case of severe (third degree) burns, since the barrier function of the skin is lost, putting the patient at risk for infection, and chronic wounds can also be fatal.

Chronic Wounds

There are three general types of chronic wounds: pressure ulcers (bedsores), venous ulcers, and diabetic ulcers. They have different causes, but the result is the same; localised tissue death. In order to treat the condition, various growth factors (cell promoters) have been tried, but so far without much success. The most favoured alternative is the use of human (or animal) skin grafts—with natural or cultured skin, or skin substitutes—the latter made from cells occurring in the human skin and in the epidermis. Other synthetic variants, such as those developed for the treatment of burns are also being investigated.

Burns

Almost all burns will heal, although the most severe will result in scarring and tissue contraction.

The treatment of severe burns entails three main requirements: getting the patient through the initial shock (which could prove fatal), eliminating fluid loss, and preventing infection. So, the ideal burn covering is skin, preferably the patient's own. Sometimes the additional trauma of a donor-site wound, or another scar on the site of the graft—elsewhere on the body—mean that surgeons have to look for alternative solutions, such as temporary skin coverings. Two temporary coverings—used while the patient gets stronger—are provided by skin taken from a cadever (allografts), or the skin from another species (xenografts), usually pig skin. Both of these have to be replaced during the healing process, as they are rejected by the immune system in a matter of days or weeks.

The FDA recognises two broad categories of wound dressing: interactive and non-interactive, and we have already considered some examples of each. In addition to a wealth of products made up from different combinations of human and animal cells, there are two currently FDA-approved interactive dressings. In order to be able to attack the problem of burns and severe chronic wounds, it would be helpful, firstly to understand the make-up and function of the skin, and what can be achieved by "Tissue Engineering".

4.2.4. *Tissue Engineering*

The skin is the body's largest organ, as well as being one of the most complex. In addition to acting as a physical barrier, it helps to control temperature through adjustments of blood flow and evaporation of sweat. It is also an important sensory organ.

Skin thickness varies with age and body location, but—in general—it averages from 1–2 mm in thickness. The skin comprises two layers: a thin outer epidermis, which is largely composed of tough, protective flat cells. When they wear away, they are replaced from underneath. The innermost part of the epidermis consists of rapidly dividing cells, called keratinocytes, which produce the tough protein keratin. The epidermis also contains a fatty substance which makes the skin waterproof.

The inner layer, the dermis, contains the skin's blood vessels, lymph vessels, nerves, hair follicles, sweat glands and oil glands. It comprises mainly connective tissue and a network of collagen protein; which gives flexibility and structure. Current approaches to tissue engineering generally fall into the following three main areas:

* Epidermal Replacement
* Dermal Replacements
* Skin Substitutes

All these techniques use cells—taken from the patient or another person—the differences being in the ways they are cultured and applied to the wound.

One product (Dermagraft, developed by Advanced Tissue Sciences and Smith & Nephew) uses a resorbable structure of polyglycolic acid and polyglactin (see Chapter 6 under resorbable sutures) seeded with collagen-forming cells (fibroblasts).

Two other products (BioBrane, marketed by Dow B Hickham) and Integra (manufactured by Integra) are worth mentioning. The former is a nylon material that contains a gelatin which interacts with clotting factors in the wound. The latter is a two-layered dressing; the top one serving as a temporary synthetic epidermis; the layer below—made from collagen fibres—acts as a lattice through which dermal tissue can begin to form.

It should be appreciated that these synthetic skins generally have to be replaced, and their function is mainly to provide a protective environment in which the body can accelerate the healing process. By this means, any subsequent skin graft will be thinner, quicker to heal, and involve less scarring.

The next stage is the provision of a synthetic skin which behaves like the real thing, including the ability the age, match pigmentation &c. Some fascinating work on the subject, with a material named "Episkin", is currently being carried out in Paris by Dr Francoise Bernard (1).

I make no apology for having devoted so much time to the understanding and treatment of chronic wounds. They provide so much misery and pain in a large proportion of the population that a solution is urgently needed. The advent of new techniques becoming available for making bioacceptable and resorbable polymers (Chapter 9) should provide a satisfying and rewarding study.

We must now consider applications where appropriately shaped materials are used to support or correct the alignment of limbs and other parts of the body

4.3. Supports

4.3.1. Rigid Supports

The simplest method of temporarily immobilising a fractured leg is to tie it to a stick, or even the other leg. A broken arm can be placed in a sling and secured to the upper body. More comfortable devices were made of wood, metal or plastic (often polypropylene); shaped to fit the limb, and padded with cotton wool, or other forms of textile.

One of the most familiar means of supporting a fractured or damaged limb, is the use of a plaster cast. This type of support is made from Plaster of Paris; a partially dehydrated form of calcium sulphate, which results from heating gypsum. Gypsum is plentiful in the Montmartre area of the Paris basin; hence the name "Plaster of Paris". When mixed with water it quickly sets to a mass of gypsum crystals, accompanied by an increase in volume. The support comes in the form of a fabric bandage, impregnated with plaster of Paris, which is moistened and wound around the area to be supported.

More sophisticated alternatives are available in the form of a knitted polyester bandage, or glass fibre tape, impregnated with a water-activated polyurethane resin. The advantages over plaster of Paris, are lightness and water resistance; since the cross-linked resin, once cured, does not react to water. The dressing is also available in a range of colours as a fashion accessory!

4.3.2. Flexible Supports

It may sometimes be necessary to provide support to a limb or part of the body, after an accident (neck brace), following an operation, or as a means of controlling pain or swelling. There is a wide range of products available for these purposes, and many of them employ very ingenious designs and combinations of materials, to allow the maximum amount of support combined with—where required—freedom of movement. The materials from which they are made include: polyester, nylon, rubbers and various metals. Fig. 4.2 shows a selection of such devices, covering various parts of the body.

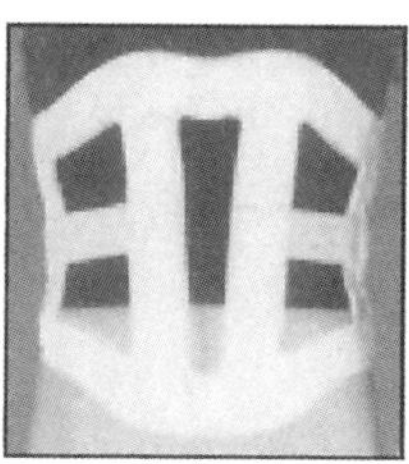
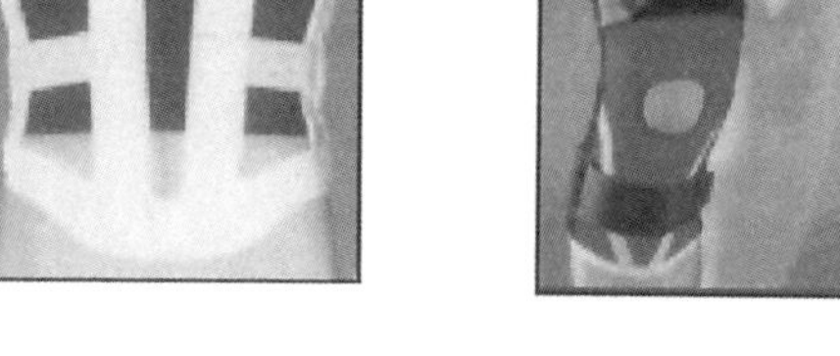
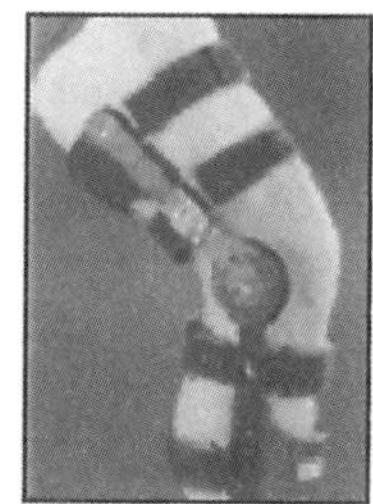

4-posr chair bace   **Knee support**   **Hinged knee brace**
                          with U-sheped patella

Figure 4.2 A selection of braces and body supports (Courtesy Luba Corporation, Seoul, Korea)

4.3.3. Corrective Supports

In this category we should distinguish between two different types:

* Passive – shapes which urge the body to adopt the correct position
* Active – those which are continually adjusted to extend or modify the required configuration

Passive Supports

These are splints or supports which, when fixed in position, are shaped so as to apply continuous pressure to the limb or part of the body, with the aim of restoring it to the desired configuration. If the correction is large, it may be necessary to carry out the correction in several stages with a succession of more aggressively shaped supports.

Active Supports

In some cases, parts of the device may be strapped to the body and the correction applied continuously either with an air pump, by means of threaded traction rods or weights (see Fig. 4.3)

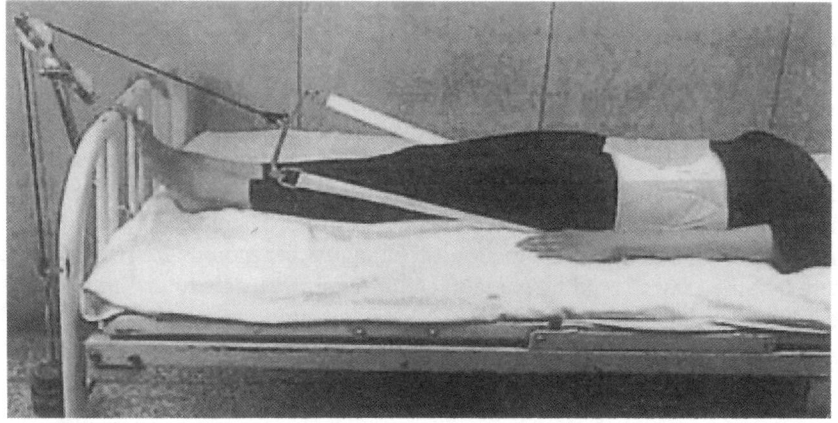

Figure 4.3 A pelvic traction belt (Courtesy Narang Enterprises, New Delhi, India)

We must make a distinction here, however, between devices which are simply applied to the body, and those in which part of the device is implanted by means of stainless steel screws (see Chapter 6). The materials used for the applications which I have described above are varied, and include: thermoplastics (polypropylene), thermosets (polyurethane), natural materials (leather, wood & cotton), glass fibre filled polyesters, aluminium and stainless steel.

We now come to an important use of materials in contact with the body, where bioacceptability and purity of materials are vital, namely: contact lenses, which are used primarily to correct a range of defects in vision, but occasionally for cosmetic effect.

4.4. Contact Lenses

4.4.1. Early Attempts

As with so many other medical applications and techniques, the history of contact lenses is a long one. The concept was first suggested in 1508 by Leonardo da Vinci (1452–1519), who made sketches of several different forms of contact lenses. Almost a hundred years later, in 1602, the French philosopher René Descartes (1596–1650) produced a more accurate description of how such a device should fit on the cornea.

In 1801, Thomas Young (1773–1829) extended Descartes' idea by using a quarter inch long (6 mm) glass tube, filled with water, and having the outer end fitted with a microscopic glass lens. A quarter of a century later, in 1827, the English astronomer, Sir John Herschel (1792–1871), suggested grinding a contact lens to conform exactly to the eye's surface.

Towards the end of the 19th century, in 1887, a German glassblower in Wiesbaden, F E Muller, created the first glass-blown lens that was designed to sit on the cornea, and—a year later, in 1888—Eugen Fick, a Swiss physician, and Eduardo Kalt, a French optometrist, almost simultaneously reported the first successful use of contact lenses to correct optical disorders. As improvements in glass technology were introduced, attempts were made—including taking moulds from living eyes—to ensure that the lenses could be made to conform more closely to the individual sclera (the fibrous coating of the eyeball). It was not until the 1930s, however, that a discovery of real significance was announced.

4.4.2. The Introduction of Plastic Contact Lenses

In 1936 Dr William Feinbloom, a New York optometrist, introduced the first successful rigid plastic contact lenses. These were made from polymethyl methacrylate (PMMA), and—at that time—were fitted with a soft, wax-like substance which hardened on the eye, so that accurate impressions of the eyeballs could be made. This technique is no longer used, since corneal curvature is now measured by highly accurate optical equipment

Although PMMA lenses gave good vision, they were initially hard to tolerate, and studies showed that—over many years—the cornea became severely altered, since the lenses did not allow the breathability, or oxygen saturation needed by the corneal cells. Although improved formulations for rigid or semi-rigid materials are now available, a development towards the end of the 1960s saw a dramatic change of direction. A Czechoslovakian chemist, Otto Wichterle, had been working with a soft, water-absorbing plastic, and this material showed considerable promise as a possible contact lens material.

4.4.3. Soft Plastic Contact Lenses

The "Wichterle" lenses, which became commercially available in 1971, were made from a material called hydroxyethylmethacrylate (HEMA). Although comfortable to wear with reduced irritation, their softness meant that they could be easily damaged. Some of the initial trials, in the United Kingdom on this type of soft lenses, were performed in 1967/68 by a research student in my own Department at Brunel University in collaboration with Mr Montague Ruben of the Moorfields Eye Hospital in London.

Over the next decade a considerable amount of work was carried out on the improvement of soft lens materials. However, because of their flexibility, soft contact lenses did not correct the oval or astigmatic cornea, although they were able to correct near- and far-sightedness, together with minimal astigmatism. This was a compromise performance which would be perfectly adequate for a majority of wearers.

Apart from the disadvantages already mentioned, the early soft contact lenses suffered from three other main defects: they absorbed proteins and bacteria from the surface of the eye—potentially a source of irritation unless the lenses were frequently removed for cleaning. They also had relatively poor oxygen transmission, which did not allow the eyes to breathe. In addition, after a few hours of continuous wear, the water-absorbing material from which they were made tended to dry out the eyes, making them tired and itchy.

4.4.4. Gas Permeable Lenses

In 1979 many of these problems were overcome by the introduction of rigid gas permeable (RGP) lenses. They were made from copolymers of PMMA and silicone elastomers, and—although called "rigid"—are much more flexible than the hard PMMA lenses, and are therefore much more comfortable to wear. In subsequent years much research was devoted to adjusting the silicone component of the copolymer so that varying degrees of wettability and oxygen transmission could be achieved. Experiments were also undertaken with coatings applied to the lens so as to reduce protein and bacteria take-up. My own company, BioInteractions Ltd., had—in the early 1990s—developed and marketed a highly effective bioacceptable coating for this purpose; but—once again—a change in direction was imminent, which would alter the concept of plastic lens-wearing.

4.4.5. Disposable Contact Lenses

In 1983, a Danish manufacturer developed a way for contact lenses to be made in a continuous wet state; a significant advance since, the material was more uniform with less distortions during manufacture. The process was acquired by Johnson & Johnson who, in 1987, introduced the first disposable contact lenses. This was followed, in 1991, by the "daily-wear two-week" replacement lenses, and—in 1995—by the "daily" disposable lenses.

These products, marketed under the trade name ACUVUE, were made from a complex polymer system called "etafilcon A", which for the scientifically minded, is a copolymer of 2-hydroxyethylmethacrylate and methacrylic acid cross-linked with 1,1,1-trimethylol propane trimethacrylate and ethylene glycol dimethacrylate, with—in the case of the daily disposable lenses—a benzotriazole UVabsorbing monomer to block the potentially harmful ultra violet radiation.

4.4.6. Comparisons & Recent Developments

There are essentially three types of contact lenses:

* Hard (PMMA) lenses, now virtually obsolete
* Soft Lenses; the most common type
* Oxygen Permeables (RGP)

Whilst improvements to the current materials and designs are constantly occurring, it might be helpful to compare the advantages and disadvantages of the last two types mentioned above, and this is done in Table 4.1.

A recent survey by Dr H Dwight Cavanagh of UT Southwestern Medical Centre in Dallas (2), showed that contact lenses, both rigid and soft, made from new high oxygen transmissible materials (silicone hydrogel and fluoro/silicone copolymers), show considerably less bacterial binding to the cornea than those currently available. In the course of the survey, three significant findings emerged:

(1) The length of wear (6 or 30 nights) appeared not to affect the amount of reduction in bacterial binding.

(2) After 6 months all soft contact lenses show enhanced lowering of bacterial binding.

(3) 30–night wear produced no significant increases in bacterial binding after one year

Finally, an unexpected finding of the study was that RGPs appear better for the eye than soft lenses, because they promote tear exchange: which washes out debris, and allows more oxygen to reach the eye.

Table 4.1 A comparison between RGP and soft lenses

Property	Oxygen Permeables (RGP)	Soft Lenses
Oxygen delivery	+++++	++
Visual acuity	+++++	++
Initial comfort	++	+++
Long term comfort	+++++	++
Durability	+++++	++
Deposit resistance	+++++	++
Cost effectiveness	+++++	++

4.4.7. A New Approach

We saw in Chapter 3 how success in achieving biocompatibility can only be truly realised if the materials we develop are virtually identical with—or make the body believe that they are—the composition and behaviour of the natural cells.

Two interesting developments along these lines have recently been reported by Carolyn Bertozzi of the Materials Sciences Division, Berkeley Lab., working with the Sunsoft Corporation (3). The first is a coating that will decrease protein binding (reducing the growth of bacteria) and at the same time increase the water binding to the surface of the lens (permitting necessary oxygen flow). The technique is summarised in Fig. 4.4.

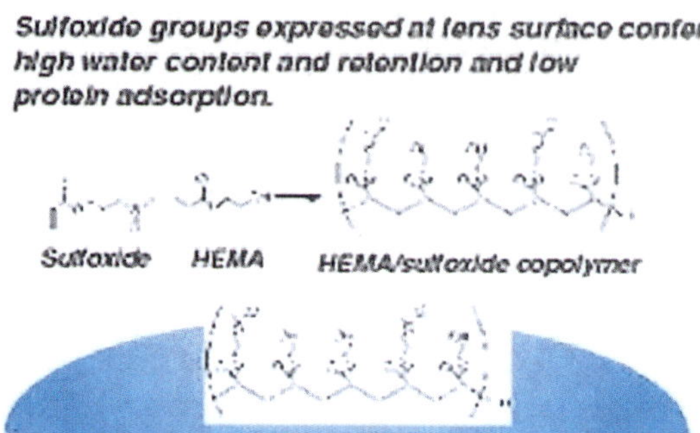

Figure 4.4 A new biocompatible contact lens material (Courtesy Carolyn Bertozzi, Berkely Lab. USA)

The second is a contact lens material that resembles the carbohydrate-coated surface of a human cell, and so binds water but not protein. This is shown schematically in Fig. 4.5.

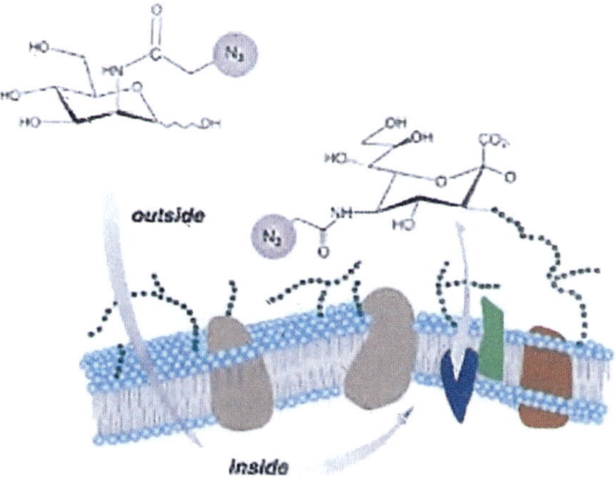

Figure 4.5 A carbohydrate hydrogel which mimics the natural cell structure of the eye (Courtesy Carolyn Bertozzi, The Berkeley Lab. USA)

Both examples employ techniques similar to those used in the BioInteractions Ltd polymers developed by Drs Sandhu & Luthra; described elsewhere in this book.

The last few years have seen many improvements in the design and manufacture of materials for contact lenses, and there will be many more. Indeed, as this chapter was being written, it was announced fromTexas Tech University, Lubbock, USA, that a team led by Dr Ted Reid had discovered that a Selenium coating only one molecule thick could considerably extend the wear time. The coating, which should stay attached to the lens for at least two years, is so thin that it does not impair oxygen transmission. It also has two main beneficial effects: it actively kills bacteria by forming chemicals called "super-peroxide radicals", and it also prevents bacterial adhesion to the cornea (4).

We should remember, however, that spectacles and contact lenses are only two of the devices and procedures for improving and maintaining the sight. Others, which involve the insertion of devices into the eye, for example: corneal grafts and retinal implants, are considered in later chapters, which deal with long term implants.

4.5. Hearing Aids

As far as this work is concerned, it is appropriate to consider hearing aids as being similar to certain types of cardiac assist devices: ie electronic equipment placed inside an inert plastic envelope. The principle difference however, is that the former— together with any leads—is worn wholly on the surface of the body. It is not necessary to concern ourselves with the internal circuitry, but the outer casing comes essentially in two forms:

* Worn inside the ear – made either of soft, silastic polymer, or from the more rigid polyurethane

* Located in the outer part of the ear, with some of the equipment behind the ear – made from a variety of materials: polyurethane, nylon or polycarbonate

In both cases, since the appliance is worn in, or against, a damp environment which is capable of harbouring infection, attempts have been made to coat the device with an anti-microbial coating of the type described in Chapter 3

4.6. Conclusion

In this chapter we have considered a number of examples where the materials— mostly plastics—are placed in contact with the body, and we have seen that in some applications—such as contact lenses and severe wound dressings—biocompatibility, and even resorption, may be of prime importance. It is interesting to note, also, that powdered glass—in the past, like silver—claimed to have curative properties, has been recently reported (December 2003) to promote healing in facial burns, when applied inside a supportive sling.

In the next chapter we shall deal with a range of applications in which the device is either inserted into the body for a relatively short time, or the body fluids—mainly blood—are passed through an extracorporeal machine: such as a kidney dialyser, or a blood oxygenator.

References

(1) Bernard F, *Laboratoires l'Oreal, Paris* (2002)
(2) Cavanagh H. Dwight, *et al, American Academy of Ophthalmology* (2001)
(3) Bertozzi C., *Biomolecular Materials Program, Berkeley Lab.* (2001)
(4) Reid E., *Texas Tech. University,* (2002)

Chapter 5

Short Term Contact Devices

5.1. Introduction

From time to time it is necessary to use devices or machines which are temporarily in contact with living tissue and blood, or other body fluids. The most commonly encountered, are catheters and drain tubes, angioplasty devices, dialysis machines, blood oxygenators (heart/lung machines), certain types of artificial hearts, other cardiac assist devices, and endotracheal and endobronchial tubes.

All of these will be expected to operate in a dynamic situation, where the nature and response of the body fluids is constantly changing, and where external factors, such as temperature, movement &c., may be expected to fluctuate. We therefore have an environment where there are two main forces in action:

* The effect of the device on the body
* The effect of the body on the device itself (see Chapter 3).

Many of the devices which I shall describe have, in their present form, evolved from the single-minded persistence of medical innovators, often with an engineering turn of mind, who were clear in their goals, and whose inventions helped to save many lives. It will thus, I think, be interesting to dwell a little on the history of the more significant developments, as well as on the present day state of the machines themselves.

5.2. Catheters

The term "catheter" is sometimes used for both catheters and drain tubes alike. However, there are differences, and I shall try to define them separately, although inevitably there will be some areas of overlap. A catheter is a tubular, generally flexible, surgical instrument that is inserted into a cavity of the body to withdraw or introduce fluid.

The most commonly encountered catheters are those used for emptying and/or irrigating the bladder. They can be inserted either through the water passage (urethral catheters), or directly into the bladder through the abdominal wall above the pubic bone (suprapubic catheters).

Catheters are made from many different materials, and the type of catheter selected depends upon the length of time the device is expected to remain in the bladder. Short-term catheters (from a few days to two weeks) are generally made from PVC or latex, while medium-term catheters (up to four weeks) are usually

85

coated with a non-irritant coating such as PTFE or silicone rubber. Exceptionally they may also be coated with a polymer which is lubricious and/or containing an anti-microbial element (see later in this chapter).

Catheters were sized on a "French" scale, according to the size of the lumen (internal diameter); the smallest on this scale being 3 French. Currently the diameter in millimetres is normally used, and a colour coding system is used to ensure that the correct size is used. A variety of different designs is available, and an inflatable balloon is incorporated in some specimens to prevent the catheter from slipping out. Some examples are shown in Fig. 5.1

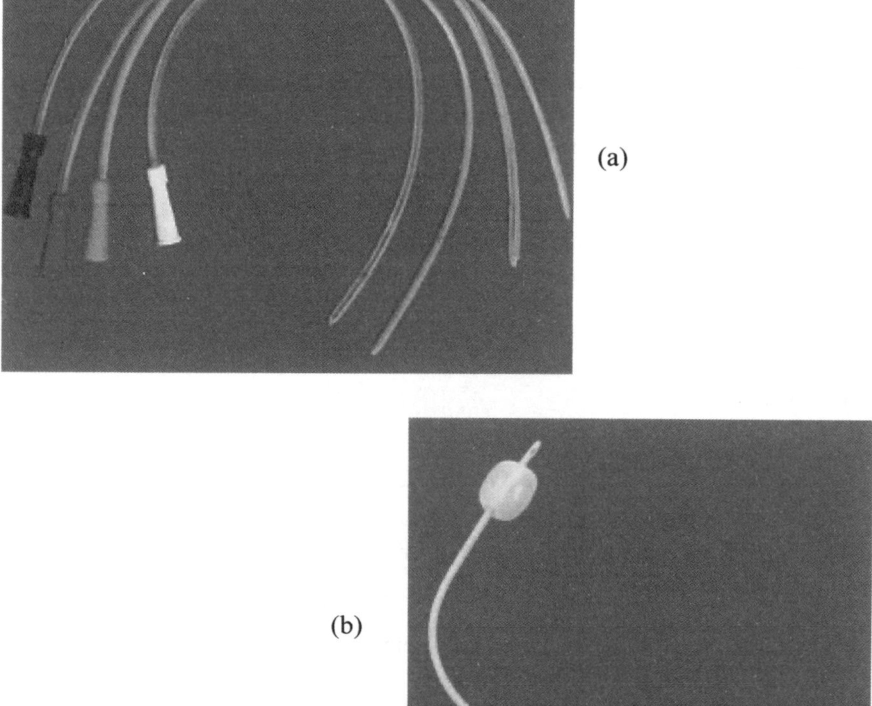

Figure 5.1 Tw types of urinary catheter (a) a short-term device (b) a Foley balloon catheter

Catheters may be also used to clear intestinal gas (flatus) and other matter from the rectum.

Within the general definition of catheters, it must be remembered that there is a range of flexible tubing used to carry out such functions as feeding through the mouth, both infants and adults, administering oxygen and anaesthetic gases through the nose, and injecting fluids through an incision (the reverse of a drain tube!).

5.3. Drain Tubes

In contrast to a catheter, a drain tube is inserted, generally into a man-made opening in the body—usually in the chest or abdomen—to drain away fluids which accumulate after an operation. As in the case of catheters, there are many different varieties of drain tubes, and it will be sufficient to give a few examples. Fig. 5.2 shows a number of different drain tubes (also sometimes known as catheters).

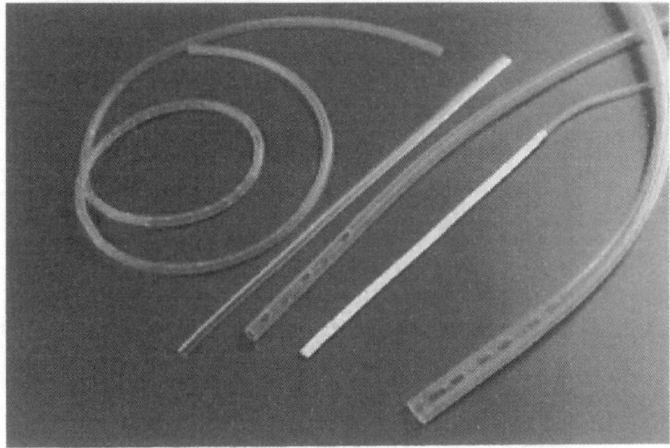

Figure 5.2 Different types of silicone rubber drain tubes

If we accept my rather arbitrary separation of the two types of intubation, we should now consider catheters (as distinct from drain tubes), and—rather confusingly also known as "cannulae"—which are inserted through an opening in the skin. These devices are know as "central venous catheters" (CVCs), and may be defined as follows. A CVC is a small biocompatible tube, or vascular access device, made of soft flexible material, which is inserted into a large vein of the peripheral vascular system. The tip of the catheter is advanced into the superior vena cava (SVC), which is located at the junction of the external jugular and sub-clavian veins in the neck. This type of catheter, of which there are many variants, is used for relatively long term therapies, including the administration of vesicant (causing blistering of the skin) drugs and chemotherapy agents.

A frequently used version of the CVC is the so-called "tunneled catheter", in which a portion of the tubing is tunneled through the subcutaneous space, and exited through the skin of the chest. Examples are the Hickman/Broviac and Groshong catheters, the latter having a simple slit valve in the tip, which remains closed in normal use; opens outwards during positive pressure (infusion or flushing), and inwards under negative pressure (drawing blood). Fig. 5.3 shows a tunneled CVC

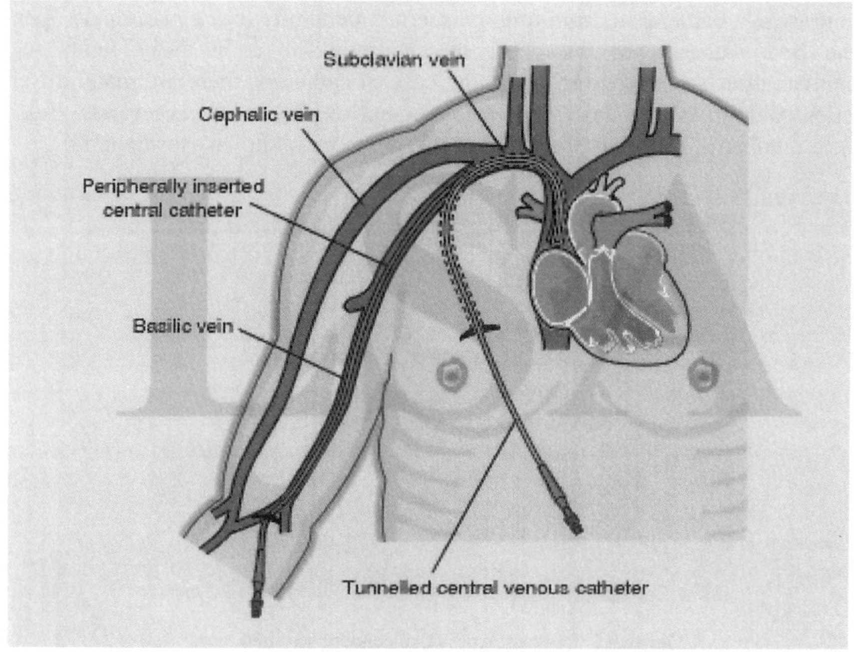

Figure 5.3 A central venous catheter

Also in this category is the PICC (peripherally inserted central catheter) line, which is inserted into a large vein in the upper arm through a break-away needle, or similar device, and the tip advanced into the SVC. This technique is not much used today in view of the danger associated with the possible migration of the needle. By a nice piece of semantics, the device is not considered to be a CVC if the tip does not terminate in the superior vena cava! Within this class of non-CVCs are epidural catheters, or cannulae, inserted into the epidural cavity (the space between the outer membrane surrounding the spinal cord and the vertebral canal) for the control of pain, and the intra-peritoneal ports, where the catheter tip is placed in the peritoneal cavity (abdomen) for drug delivery.

Within the general definition of catheters we must also briefly mention implanted venous access devices, which comprise a silicone catheter attached to a self-sealing septum—encased in a titanium, plastic or steel port—which is placed in a subcutaneous pocket, generally in the arm. The tip of the catheter is located in the SVC, and the other end is tunneled under the skin and attached to the port. An alternative method is to attach the port to the surface of the arm instead of implanting it.

Two further catheter variants are the endotracheal tube and the endobronchial tube. When inserted into the lung, double-lumen endotracheal tubes serve to isolate ventilation, separating the right and left pulmonary units—using two separate endotracheal tubes. In the latter case, endobronchial tubes—used in thoracic surgery—employ two inflaable balloons, or cuffs, to seal off the bronchus and trachea as required. Fig. 5.4 shows a double-lumen endobronchial tube.

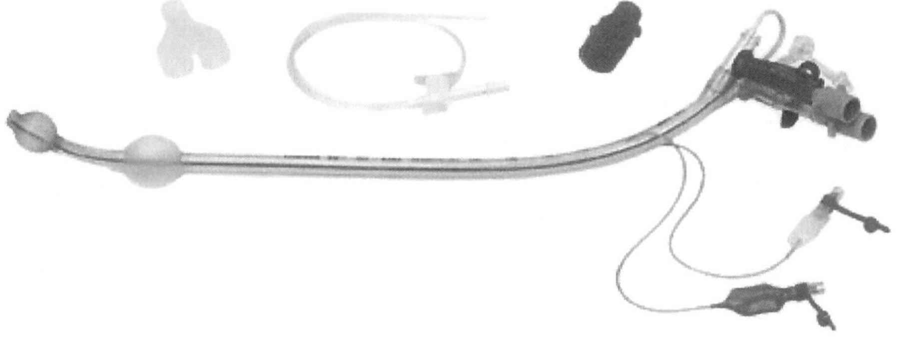

Figure 5.4 A Portex double-limen endobronchial tube (Courtesy Smiths Medical, London, England)

Even from this brief introduction to catheters and drain tubes, it is evident that there are numerous different combinations of tubes and attachments, and that many different materials may be involved in their production. It is also apparent that for such a diversity of applications, the "normal" characteristics of materials need to be modified. Thus we find that special polymeric coatings have been devised, by a British Company (BioInteractions Ltd) which confer a greater degree of lubricity (slipperiness) for ease of insertion; and also others which change their mechanical properties: allowing the tube to be flexible for insertion, and less so when in situ (1).

These and other "memory" phenomena are discussed in Chapter 10. Meanwhile, Table 5.1 summarises some of the materials used for catheters, cannulae and drain tubes.

Table 5.1 Materials used in catheters and drain tubes

Device type	Material	Description
Central venous catheters	Silicone rubber	Soft
	Polyurethane PTFE	Stiffer than Silicone, used in triple lumen catheters
	Elastomeric hydrogel	Stiff when dry, softens, extends and expands when *wet*
	Polyester	Cuff just below exit to hold catheter in place, and prevent infection
Venous access devices	Silicone rubber	Used for caheter/cannula
	Titanium Steel Polyurethane Epoxy	Used for body of device

5.4. Angioplasty Devices

Angioplasty may be defined as the surgical repair or reconstruction of a narrowed or completely blocked blood vessel, usually an artery; less commonly a vein. In percutaneous transluminal angioplasty (PTA, balloon angioplasty) an inflatable balloon, mounted on the tip of a flexible catheter, is inserted through the skin and placed within the lumen (the space within a tubular or sac-like part, such as a blood vessel, the intestine, or the stomach) of the affected artery, and guided to the blockage under X-ray screening control. The balloon is then inflated, compressing the accumulated plaque against the intima (the inner wall of the artery). This disruption of the intima by the applied pressure of the balloon, not only restores the channel through the vessel, but appears to delay the onset of restenosis (the return of the arterial narrowing).

Although angioplasty is successful in re-opening the arteries, there is often a tendency for restenosis to occur after a while, and for the channel through the centre of the artery to narrow again. A number of treatments were tried, including the use of laser angioplasty in the early 1980s. These efforts were met with some success, largely as a result of the refinements in laser fibre-optics, and the procedure is now used for clinical recanalisation in both coronary and peripheral arteries.

As well as simply enlarging the bore of the artery by balloon angioplasty, it is now common to complement this technique by the insertion of a mechanical device called a "stent". Stents are small expandable cylinders—generally made of metal or plastics—which are carried on the tip of the catheter, implanted in the artery in the collapsed state, and expanded in situ by inflating the balloon, to keep the passage open. It will be recalled that when we were considering thoracic surgery (Chapter 1), we saw that stents were used with synthetic aortic replacements in order to keep them open .

In order to carry out their desired role effectively stents must satisfy a number of requirements, which include:

<u>Mechanical</u>

* Flexibility   * Low unconstrained profile
* High radial strength   * Reliable expansion habit
* Radio opaque   * Trackable

<u>Flow</u>

* Biocomptibility   * Thromboresistant
* Hydrodynamically compatible   * Circumferential coverage

There are also many different designs of stents, but they may be grouped into the following four principal categories:

* Wire mesh
* Wire coil
* Tubular slotted
* Continuously connected (expanded metal type)

Although the use of open-work designs for stents makes it possible for the device to be surrounded by body tissue, thus reducing the likelihood of rejection, nevertheless—in some 25% of cases—the formation of scar tissue causes the arterial lumen to again become narrowed. Coating with an immunosuppressive drug helps to minimise this reaction, and considerable research is continuing in the use of coatings which are anti-thrombogenic. Trials have been made to develop a coating which releases an appropriate drug continuously into the bloodstream.

Other techniques are being developed to progressively eliminate, stents. For example, experiments with biodegradable plastic stents have been carried out in Japan (2). Also, since even the presence of the plastic stent can cause a degree of rejection, it is planned to incorporate anti-inflammatory drugs into the plastic coils, which could be delivered right into the arteries while the coils dissolve. Self-expanding stents, made of special alloys that expand over time inside the artery also look promising, as does the recently tried technique of coating the inside of the artery with a special polymer which hardens, forming a smooth "pavement" inside it.

Interestingly enough, it was recently reported (3) that the use of beta radiation had resulted in a reduction of restenosis in patients whose arteries had been kept open by the use of stents. Fig. 5.5 shows a number of different metal stent profiles.which have been evaluated by Drs Ruygrok & Serruys (4).

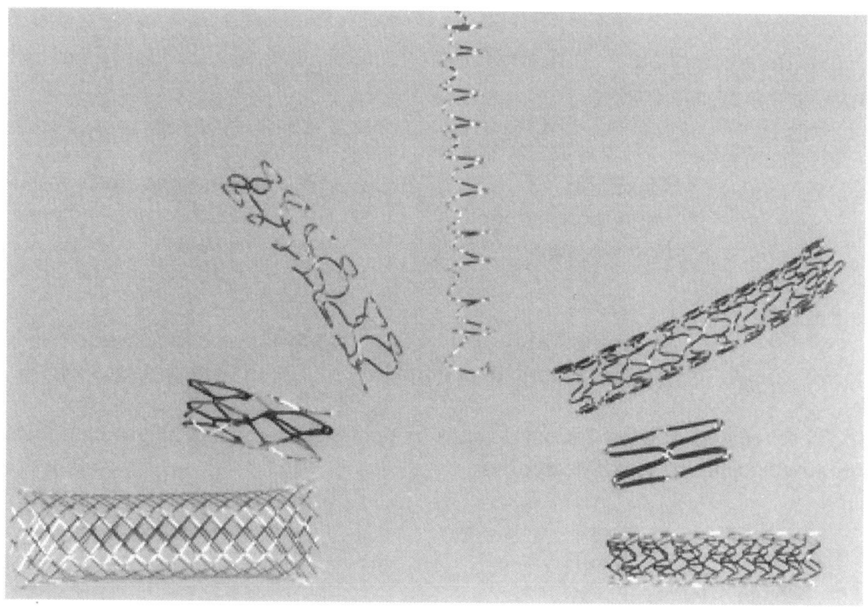

Figure 5.5 Stent patterns; clockwise from left to right; (1) Wallstent (2) Palmer-Schatz stent (3) Wiktor stent (4) Gianturco-Roubin stent (5) Cordis stent (6) AVE stent (7) Multilink stent

Of the large variety of stents, and stent delivery systems, currently available, two are worth lookng at, and are shown in Fig. 5.6.

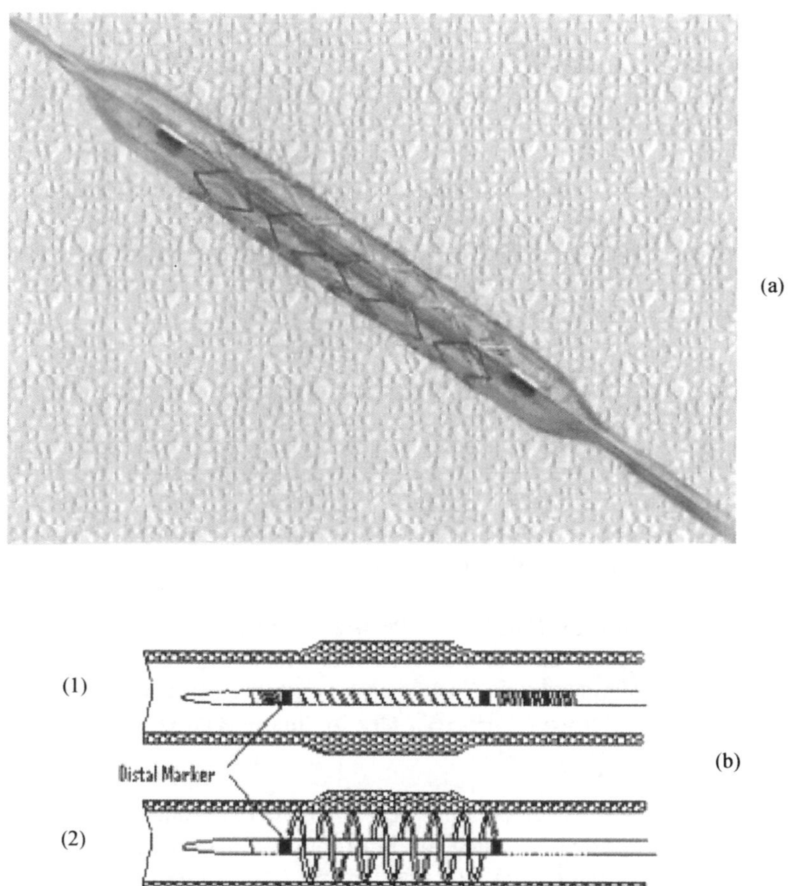

Figure 5.6 Stent types; (a) The Perico peripheral stent inside the plastic delivery balloon (b) The IntraCoil[R] self-expanding peripheral stent with delivery sheath (1) before release and (2) after release

Having regard to what has already been said about stents and their performance requirements, the development of new materials is an important facet of stent technology. The most commonly used materials include stainless steel, tantalum, nitinol (nickel and titanium alloys) and platinum, with some gold for radio-opacity. Polymeric materials with the right mechanical characteristics—such as polyamides— have been used, but the problem of overcoming their transparency to radiation (for tracking) has still to be overcome. A variety of coating materials, including PTFE, have been used with metal stents to improve their biocompatibility (the use of coatings to reduce the effects of rejection was covered in Chapter 3).

5.5. Extra-Corporeal Machines

5.5.1. Kidney Dialysis Machines

When the kidneys are no longer able to carry out their function of cleaning and maintaining the blood, several remedies are available. If the loss of kidney function is permanent, as in ESRD (End Stage Renal Disease), the most likely treatment would be to consider a kidney transplant (Chapter 1). However, where the damage is less severe, dialysis offers an alternative.

The Principles of Dialysis

This treatment cleans the blood, and removes waste and excess water from the body, as is normally done by the healthy kidneys. Sometimes dialysis is a temporary procedure, but—when renal failure is severe and permanent—it will be necessary for the treatment to be carried out on a regular basis.

In 1861, Thomas Graham (1805–869) Professor of Chemistry at St Andrew's University in Glasgow, observed that dissolved solids (solutes) were able to diffuse through a semi-permeable membrane (in this case vegetable parchment coated with albumin). He called the process "dialysis", and by this means was able to extract urea from urine.

Although partially successful attempts were made in 1913, and again in 1924, to produce an "artificial kidney"—using hirubin (obtained from leach heads) as an anticoagulant—it was not until the 1940s that heparin (an anticoagulant discovered in 1922, and used to prevent clotting of blood samples) was used as a systemic anticoagulant in humans. This led to the development in 1944 of the first practical human haemodialysis machine, by Willem Kolff (1911–   ), who was living in German occupied Holland during World War II.

Early Dialysis Machines

The device. illustrated in Fig. 5.7, comprised a rotating drum or barrel made from wooden slats with open spaces between them. Round the drum were wound some 30-40 metres of cellophane "sausage" casing, through which the blood was "pumped" by means of the patient's heart and blood pressure. The lower half of the drum rotated in a bath containing the dialysis liquid, which removed the impurities in the blood. Metal or glass tubes were used to complete the circuit through an artery and vein. Although the machine worked satisfactorily, such a large volume of blood was required to circulate outside the body, that blood transfusion was required.

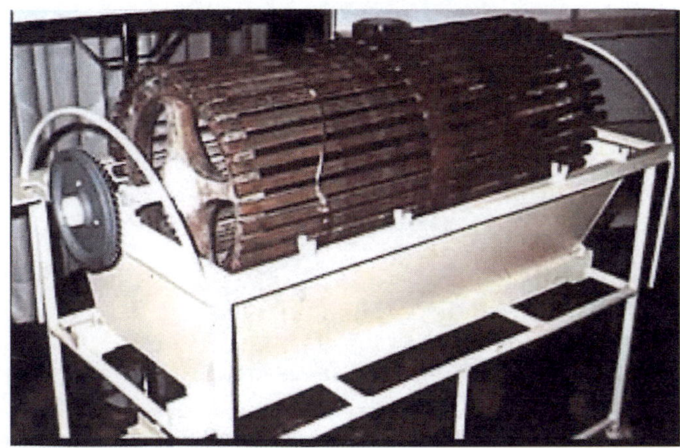

Figure 5.7 One of Kolff's first dialysis machines

After the war Kolff migrated to the United Sates, and continued his work, which resulted in the introduction of a "twin coil" dialyser, in which the cellophane tubing was wound round a vertically mounted drum, a development of the concept originally put forward in 1946 by Nils Alwell (see Fig. 5.8).

One of the main problems in treating patients with acute renal failure was the need to get adequate flows of blood into the dialysis machine, and the access methods used—glass or metal tubes, which could only be used once per pair of blood vessels—tended to exhaust veins and arteries very quickly, with the result that only a few dialysis treatments could be undertaken. It as not until the mid 1950s, when teflon (PTFE) and silastic (silicone rubber) were developed, that the first "safe" long lasting, flexible blood access became possible.

Nowadays the most common way of providing permanent access to the bloodstream is to create an internal fistula in the arm. This involves having an artery and a vein connected surgically. When they are joined, the stronger blood flow from the artery causes the vein to expand; needles can then be inserted into the enlarged vein for connection to the dialyser. An alternative method is to insert an internal graft. In this procedure an artery is connected to the vein with a short piece of synthetic tubing placed under the skin. Needles can be inserted into the graft for connection to the dialyser.

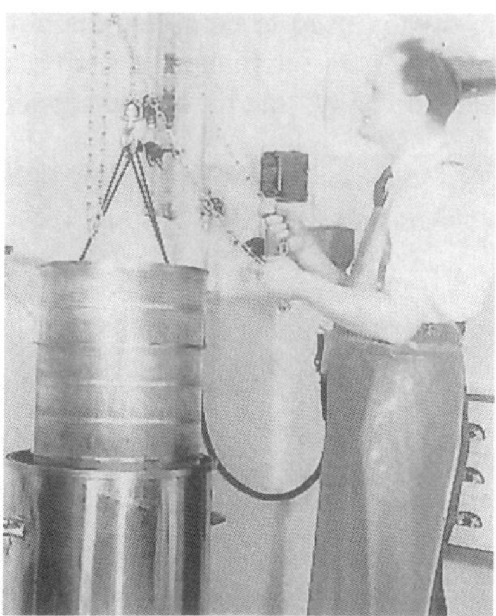

Figure 5.8 The Alwall dialyser in the 1950s. The tubing is wound round a vertically mounted screed (Courtesy Dr N Hoenich)

The development of techniques to use blood vessels repeatedly, while preserving them, made it possible to keep patients with permanent renal failure alive for longer periods, and the growth of renal units began. The first outpatient haemodialysis centre was established in Seattle, USA in 1962.

Improvements in the Design of Dialysis Machines

The coil dialysers had a number of performance defects, including the inability to produce uniform dialysate flow across the membrane, and several important modifications were introduced. The first was the parallel plate dialyser, in which membrane sheets—mounted on plastics support screens—were stacked in layers, ranging from 2–20 or more. In this system the blood and dialysate are able to travel through a series of multiple parallel channels with very little resistance to flow.

The next improvement to take place was the introduction of hollow fibres in place of the flat or tubular membrane. The fibres, made from polysulphone, were embedded in a polyurethane plug contained in the tube sheet The blood passed through the centre of the hollow fibres, and the dialysate was pumped around them. Latterly the assembly was produced in the form of a disposable cartridge which fitted into the polycarbonate casing.

These advances were matched not only in the design of dialysis machines, but also in the procedure of dialysis itself. Fig. 5.9 shows a parallel plate dialyser, and Fig. 5.10 illustrates the the principles of the more modern hollow fibre system.

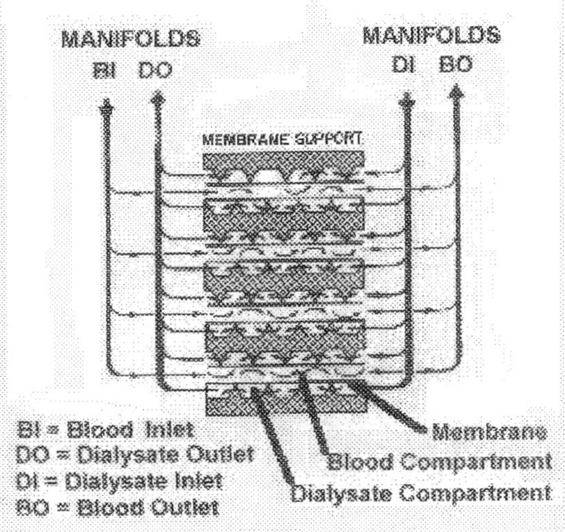

Figure 5.9 A parallel plate dialyser

Currently, the extracted blood is pumped simultaneously with the dialysis solution, while the machine monitors both circuits, and adjusts the composition of the dialysis solution while adding coagulants to the blood, to prevent clotting.

At the same time the machine removes the water which healthy people eliminate via the kidneys. Nowadays it is common for more water than strictly necessary to be filtered out, as this increases the effectiveness of the cleansing process. To compensate for this fluid loss the patient is simultaneously given an infusion.

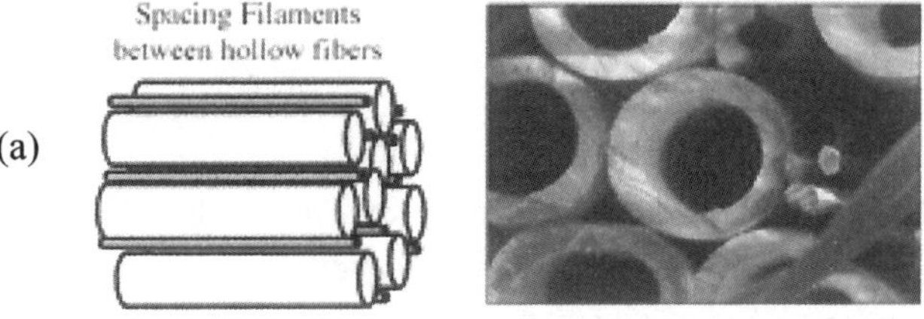

     Life-enhancing Plastics

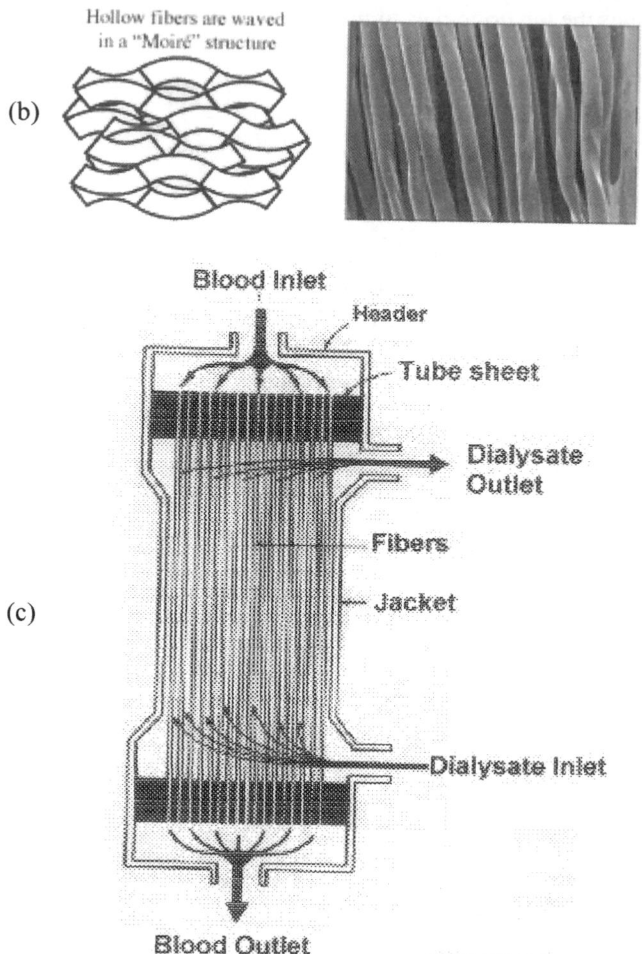

Figure 5.10 A hollow fibre dialyser, (a) & (b) diferent configurations of the fibres (c) a cross-section through the fibre container

The fibre configurations are described in an outline of the course syllabus on the Advances in Nephrology and Dialysis, Vicenza, Italy (5).

So "patient friendly" has the process become, that many cruise liners, and also holiday resorts are offering dialysis facilities for people on holiday.

Fig. 5.11 illustrates a modern dialysis circuit, and also shows a dialysis unit overlooking the bay in Bodrum, Turkey.

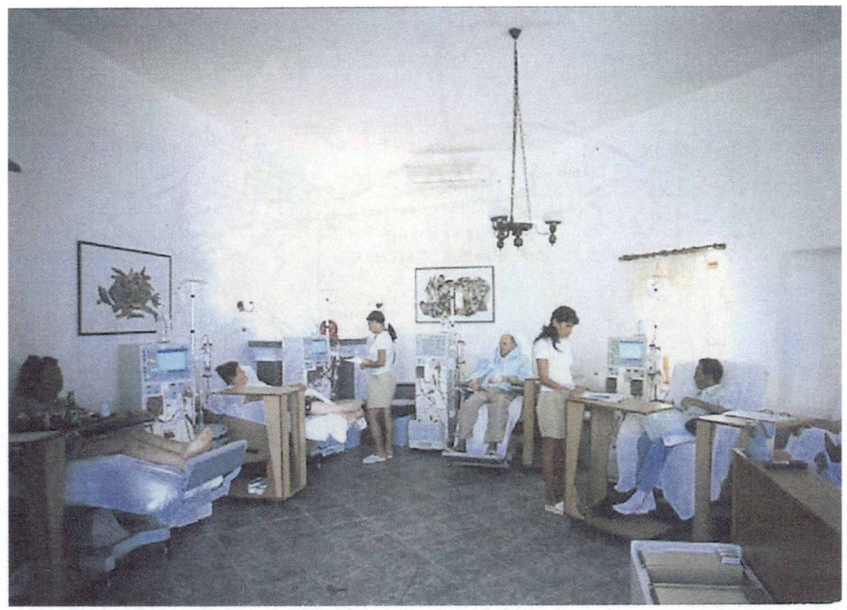

Figure 5.11 The dialysis suite at Bodrum (Courtesy Medical & Dialysis Center, Bodrum , Turkey)

In parallel with these developments in hospital dialysis, home dialysis was introduced in the mid 1960s, to overcome the difficulties in providing adequate facilities for the increasing number of patients, as well as to allow treatment without a hospital visit. Interestingly enough, one of the first home dialysis systems was set up in Japan, in 1961, using a domestic washing machine. Fig. 5.12 shows the layout of this ingenious idea..

For completeness we should now consider very briefly two other types of kidney dialysis. These are: slow continuous renal replacement therapy, and peritoneal dialysis.

Haemodialysis Systems

The first was devised in an attempt to improve the treatment of acute renal failure in critically ill patients under intensive care, and comprises four related techniques.

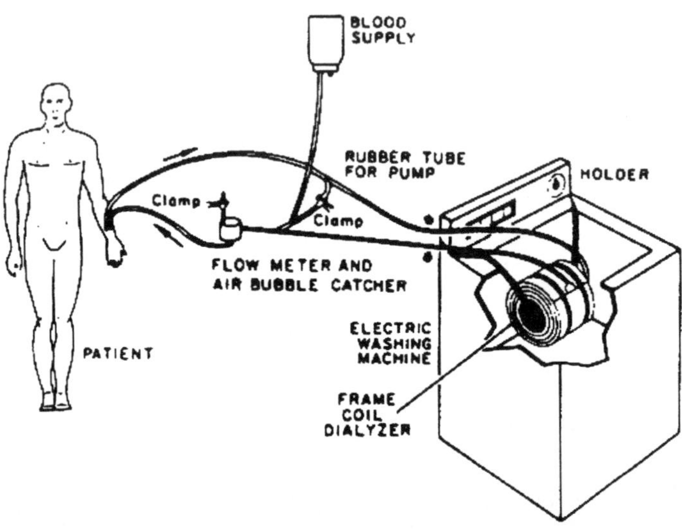

Figure 5.12 A Japanese home dialysis system using a domestic washing machine. It functions like the Kolff-Travenol machine (Courtesy the Renal Unit, the Royal Infirmary, Edinburgh, Scotland)

Continuous arteriovenous haemofiltration (CAVH) is accessed through the femoral artery and vein, and the blood is passed through a small hollow fibre haemofilter. Heparin is infused continuously, by means of a pump, into the arterial line.

Continuous venovascular haemofiltration ((CVVH) is pump assisted, and—because of its higher throughput—is replacing CAVH. Access is achieved by means of a double lumen catheter inserted in the femoral, subclavian, or internal jugular vein. Dialysis is carried out by infusing a dialysis fluid as a counter current to the blood.

The third technique, Continuous arteriovenous haemodialysis (CAVHD) uses a set-up similar to CAVH, but uses the blood/dialysate interface as the haemodialysis membrane.

Finally, Continuous arteriovenous haemodialysis (CAVHD) uses an infusion pump, haemodialysis membrane and dialysate solution as well as the same access circuitry as the CVVH process. As with the CAVHD system, adding the dialysis membrane and the dialysate solution increases the efficiency of the process.

Peritoneal Dialysis

An alternative to haemodialysis is peritoneal dialysis, which employs the peritoneal membrane itself to separate impurities from the blood, and is used with blood access in the abdomen. In the early stages it was necessary to insert a catheter into the abdomen each time dialysis took place.

This had the disadvantages that the catheter had to be inserted under local anaesthetic, and the use of an in-dwelling catheter carried the risk of infection. The development of a soft (silastic) tunnelled catheter that could be left in place, made peritoneal dialysis a viable treatment

Materials used in Dialysis

As we have seen, quite a wide range of materials, many of them plastics, are used in the process of dialysis, and a brief summary is given below.

Membranes – Natural and synthetic materials are used, including: regenerated cellulose (both irradiated and 'plain'), cellulose esters, polysulphone. polyacrylonitrile, polymethyl methacrylate and polyvinylidene fluoride.

Accessories – Polycarbonate, polyamide, polyurethane, polypropylene, glass beads and a variety of steels and metal alloys.

The material is only one of the parameters in dialyser manufacture. Also important are the design of the flow paths, and the processing history of the different components. Also, since the blood passes through a system with changes in materials, as well as in geometry, the remarks in Chapter 3 relating to blood damage and clotting are of particular relevance, and much of the blood path has to be treated with an appropriate biocompatible coating.

5.5.2. *The Heart-Lung Machine — Blood Oxygenator*

The function of the heart-lung machine, is to divert the patient's blood from the heart, so as to allow the surgeon to operate on the damaged heart. The blood is removed by means of a tube inserted into the right-hand side of the heart, and pumped through an oxygenator, which replicates the action of the lungs by removing carbon dioxide and replacing oxygen. It is then returned "downstream" into the left-hand side. When the patient is 'on bypass' the temperature of the blood is often cooled from its normal level of about 37^0C to about 30^0C, which reduces the need for oxygen, and consequently the work that the machine has to do.

Early Developments

In 1931, the American Surgeon John Gibbon, had watched a patient struggle for life after an emergency operation. Gibbon said that "During the long night's vigil.....the thought occurred to me that the patient's life might be saved if the blue blood in her veins could be continuously withdrawn into an extra-corporeal blood circuit, exposed to an atmosphere of oxygen, and then returned to the patient by way of a systemic artery." In his imagination Gibbon had conceived the essence of the heart-lung machine, but it took nearly two decades to build it.

In order to achieve what Gibbon had imagined, such a machine must be mechanically reliable, able to be operated by hand in the event of power failure, and so constructed that all components are repairable without risk to the patient. In addition to the relatively obvious needs just mentioned, it is also necessary for the following important requirements to be met:

* Must not damage the blood
* Must allow flow and pressure to be adjusted according to changing needs
* Must allow alterations in temperature to be carried out
* Must allow efficient gas exchange at all temperatures and flow rates

What we are looking for, therefore, is a box—as small as possible to avoid the need to prime, or top-up, with large amounts of fluid—into which the blood is driven, as gently as possible past a membrane—or stack of membranes—through which the exchange of gases (O_2 and CO_2) with the blood can take place.

The circuit through which the blood travels must be smooth, without sharp changes in profile, and minimal mechanical movement (valves, taps &.) So as to offer minimal potential damage to the blood. The pump, too, must not crush the blood or generate turbulence. The pumps currently in use are either developments of the roller and the principle devised by Michael DeBakey (1908-   ) in his early pioneering work on open heart surgery, or of the centrifugal type.

Later Developments

Despite early setbacks, and discouragement from colleagues, Gibbon persisted in his experiments and, in 1935, he used a prototype heart-lung bypass machine to keep a cat alive for 26 minutes.

After war service in the Far East, Gibbon resumed his work and, in 1953, a patient, Cecelia Bavolek, became the first person successfully to undergo open heart bypass surgery. The machine, which used a novel method of cascading the blood down a permeable membrane, totally supported her heart and lung function for more than half the operation.

In 1952, the Swedish physician, Viking Olov Bjork, invented an oxygenator with multiple screen discs that rotated slowly in a shaft over which a film of blood was injected. Oxygen was passed over the rotating discs, and the device was successfully used on a human patient a Stokholm's Soder Hospital in 1954. Later versions of the machine improved the biocompatibility of the system by having a silicone lining throughout the system, which helped to delay clotting and minimise damage to the platelets.

We have already seen that, as in the case of kidney dialysis machines (discussed earlier in this chapter), the first gas exchange devices were semi-permeable plastic membranes, and in the 1960s silicone elastomers were found to be capable of transporting oxygen more than 50 times more efficiently than other currently available materials. Their ability to transport CO_2 at least 6 times better than O_2 also came very close to the body's natural requirements. Fig. 5.13 shows Dr (later Professor) Nora Burns engaged in the manufacture of a polydimethylsiloxane membrane as a continuous web. The machine and extrusion process were developed in my own laboratories at Brunel University.

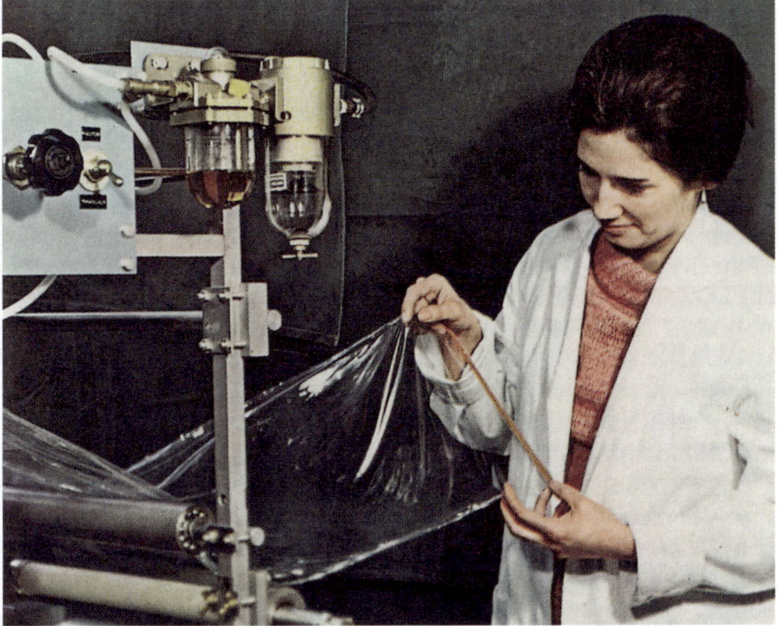

Figure 5.13 The production of a silicone elastomer membrane at the Royal Postgraduate Medical School in London (Courtesy Aldus Books)

Despite the success of these early developments, it was soon realised that membrane systems were relatively inefficient in their ability to bring the bulk of the red cells contained in a sample of blood to the surface of the membrane, so as to effect an efficient gas exchange. Increasing the surface area of the membrane assembly by stacking successive sheets while massaging the blood between the sheets with bubbles of oxygen, gave some improvement, but added to the complexity of the system, as well as the potential for blood damage.

An alternative was to adopt the method of the heat exchanger, found in cars and steam railway engines, whereby a fluid is passed through a series of interconnecting tubes over which a stream of air is passed. Fig. 5.14 shows such a system made by Medtronic Inc.

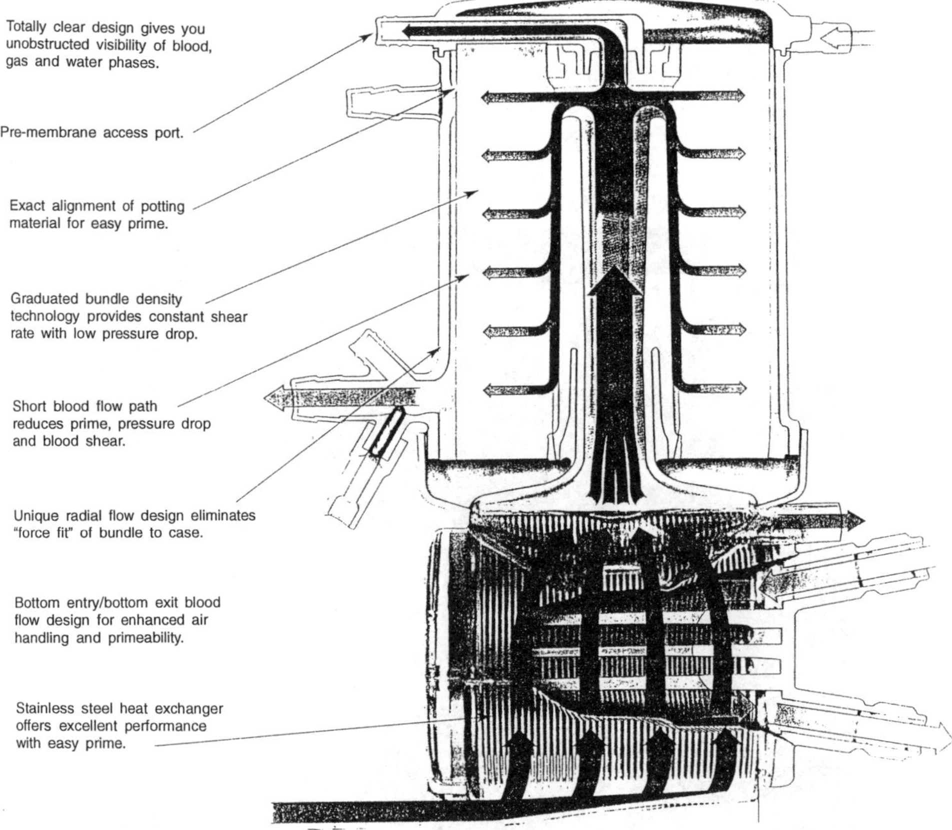

Fig. 5.14 The gas exchange system of a modern blood oxygenator (Courtesy Medtronic Inc.)

An alternative is to pass the gas through the hollow fibres, which are surrounded by the blood.

The device shown in Fig. 5.14 operates in much the same way as the modern dialysis machines already described, except that in the latter there are two liquid circuits. In the case of the blood oxygenator ilustrated in Fig. 5.14, the bundle of hollow propylene fibres—together with all other internal surfaces—is coated with a biocompatible coating (Trillium Biopassive Surface™), developed by my own company. BioInteractions Ltd. for Medtronic Inc. (6). This coating contains an anticoagulant (heparin) together with other specific chemical groupings designed to minimise protein and cell deposition. In addition to containing the means of exchanging gases, the oxygenator is provided with a stainless steel heat exchanger to ensure that the blood is maintained at the correct temperature throughout the period on bypass. The transparent housing is made from polycarbonate.

It should also be mentioned that, in addition to the heart-lung machines already discussed, there is a range of portable devices and ventilator systems, which embody many of the elements of the "full-size" machines.

5.6. Conclusion

In this chapter we have covered a wide range of applications in which the materials of the various devices come into temporary, or short term, contact with the body fluids. In some cases the device is inserted into the body—either through a natural orifice, or one that has been created—in others the fluids have been removed from the body and circulated outside it through a machine. We must now turn to procedures in which devices are inserted, or implanted, into the body for somewhat longer periods.

References

(1) Luthra A.K & Sandhu S S, *Medical Device Technology*, Oct. pp 10–16 (2002)
(2) Tamai H & Igaki K, *Circulation,* 102, pp 371–3, 399–404 (2000)
(3) Marks D S, *Healthlink (Wisconsin),* 7 Dec. (2001)
(4) Serruys P W et al (ed), *Handbook of Coronary Stents,* 3rd Edition, Martin Dunitz Publishing Ltd. (2000)
(5) Ronco C, Ghezzi P M & Guiseppi La G, *Journal of Nephrology,* 12, (Suppl 2), pp S68–S81 (1999)
(6) Luthra A K & Sandhu S S, US Patent 6,096,798 (2000)

Chapter 6

Medium Term Implants

6.1. Introduction

In this chapter I propose to deal with a number of material applications where the devices are implanted into the body for a relatively short period of time. They are then either removed, or tend to become absorbed by the body once their function has been completed. Obvious examples of the former include plates and traction devices, which are used either to ensure that fractured bones may complete their healing process in the correct alignment, or where it may be necessary to extend the length of a bone. The latter categories include such topics as soluble stitches, and the biodegradable "scaffolding" used to promote organ growth (see Chapter 10).

I have also made the rather arbitrary decision to include mechanical hearts in this discussion, since it can be argued that they should be included in Chapter 7 with pacemakers &c. However, they were originally intended to serve only until a donor heart became available. Also, current experience with "permanent" implantation, although encouraging, is still very recent and cannot yet provide any reliable data.

6.2. The Mechanical Heart

In many cases, heart disease may be so advanced that there is no chance of the patient surviving until a suitable donor heart can be located. Therefore, in the early 1950s, medical scientists and engineers set out to design a device that would keep the patient alive for the intervening period. Although in this search, a wide variety of different solutions was produced, and the principles often overlapped, the methods of treatment resolved themselves into two main categories:

* Artificial Hearts – Taking over the function of the whole heart
* Ventricular Assist Devices – Helping the damaged part of the heart to function

6.2.1. Artificial Hearts

The credit for inventing the first artificial heart must go to Willem Kolff (see Chapter 1), who became interested in cardiovascular problems during his seventeen year stay at the Cleveland Clinic Foundation, in Ohio, USA. While there, he also invented the intra-aortic balloon pump, to help maintain circulation during heart attacks. This device, later improved by Dr Adrian Kantrowitz, will be discussed later in this chapter. In 1957 Kolff designed a mechanical heart, powered by an external electrical supply, which was implanted in a dog who survived for 90 minutes. Later, a calf was implanted with a Kolff heart, and the animal survived for 31 hours.

In 1969, a team of researchers led by Dr Denton A Cooley of the Texas Heart Institute, performed the world's first total artificial heart (TAH) implant. The "heart", designed by Dr Domingo Liotta, was able to keep the patient alive for more than 60 hours until a donor heart became available for transplantation. The device (shown in Fig. 6.1) was an air-driven double-ventricle pump, connected to the power unit by silastic tubing covered by Dacron (polyester) fabric.

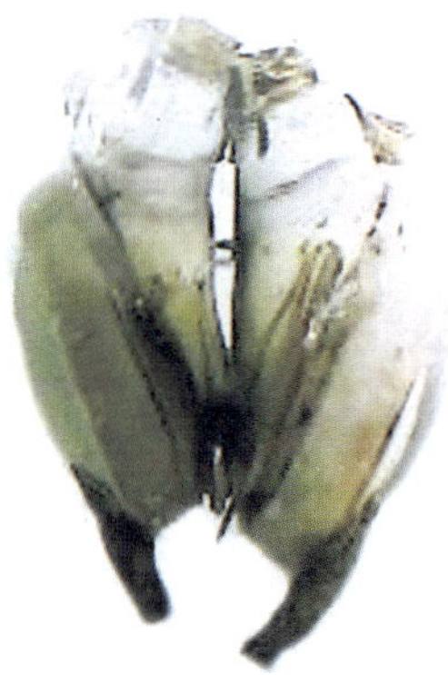

Figure 6.1 The Liotta Total Artificial Heart, (Courtesy the Texas Heart Institute, USA)

The blood flow through the device was controlled by hinge-less valves. The two pump chambers (the "ventricles") were made from silastic polymer and Dacron fabric, and the cuff-shaped inflow tracts (the "atria") as well as the outflow tracts were made of Dacron fibre, covered with Dacron velour to encourage smooth cellular growth.

In the next decade or so, work was concentrated mainly on the development of a permanently implantable device, and—in 1981—Denton Cooley implanted a second machine (developed by Dr Tetsuzo Akutzu) which kept the patient alive for 55 hours until a donor heart was found. The pumping chambers were one-piece mouldings from Avothane (a smooth-finished polyurethane), and the inflow and outflow ports contained Björk-Shiley disc valves (see Chapter 7). The prosthetic ventricles were attached to the natural heart's atria, and major blood vessels, by flexible silastic tubes. The pumps were connected to the external electrical and pneumatic power console by Dacron velour-covered tubing. The Akutzu heart is shown in Fig 6.2(a).

In 1982, twenty-five years after his experiment with the dog, Kolff and Dr William De Vries of the University of Utah, used an aluminium and polyurethane air-powered heart (the Jarvik–7), designed by Dr Robert Jarvik, to replace the diseased hearts of four patients. The first was a 61 year old dentist, Dr Barney Clark. After mechanical failures on the operating table, he survived for 112 days; four months of suffering that included convulsions, renal failure, respiratory problems, mental disturbance and multi-organ failure. The second patient, William Schroeder, lived for 18 months, despite multiple strokes and haemorrhages, and the FDA promptly shut the project down. Fig. 6.2(b) illustrates the Jarvik–7 artificial heart.

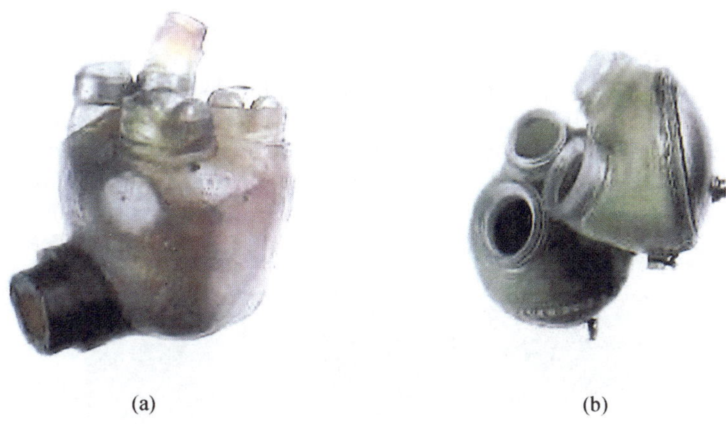

(a)   (b)

Figure 6.2 Two early examples of TAHs (a) the Akutzu III model (b) the Jarvik–7, (Courtesy the Texas Heart Institute, USA)

After a time, surgeons found that the Jarvik–7, when used extra-corporeally, could be used as a temporary bridge to a heart transplant, and kept some patients alive for several months until a new heart could be found.

Although the device was intended to bridge the gap until donor organs became available, it must be remembered that, in all the early mechanical heart cases, the patients were obliged to remain tethered to a console about the size of a domestic washing machine, which severely restricted their mobility and quality of life.

Despite these setbacks, Robert Jarvik was determined, along with others, to press on with the development of a more compact and reliable device which could, ideally, be programmed and powered (or recharged) from outside the body. The need for connections, tubes or wires, to pass through the skin, was not only an inconvenience, but a possible source of infection. Jarvik also turned his attention to the improvement of ventricular assist devices, which we shall consider in the next section.

Building a mechanical heart is a very complex task. The pump's diaphragm, bladders—or other means of transmission—must flex some 40 million times a year, have to pump faster or slower according to the changing needs of the body, must fit within the chest cavity, be resistant to the effects of the body fluids and infection, must not cause blood clotting, and must work for very long periods without lubrication or maintenance. Many of these requirements are now within our reach, thanks to the engineering achievements of the aerospace industry.

In order to ensure that the different components are disposed within the body in the most effective way, before surgery is attempted, the patient receives a standard MRI or CAT scan, which is translated into a three-dimensional colour model of the prospective patient. Ultimately, after some 30 years of research, an American company, Abiomed Inc., from Massachussetts, and its collaborators, with the support of the National Heart Lung and Blood Institute, came up with the first entirely self-contained implantable heart, the AbioCor, which was successfully inserted into a patient in the sumer of 200. Fig. 6.3 shows the AbioCor Replacement heart

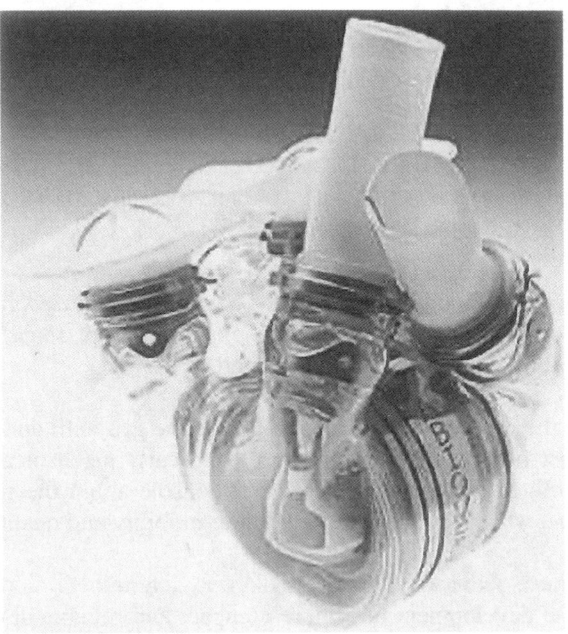

Figure 6.3 The AbioCor Replacement Heart, (Courtesy Abiomed Inc., Massachussetts, USA)

The AbioCor consists of an internal thoracic unit, comprising a two-chambered titanium electric pump using flexible plastic bladders to drive blood through the body, and self-contained rechargeable battery, a miniaturised electronics package, power transfer coil, and an internally worn battery package. The device's batteries can be recharged by means of the wireless energy transfer system, which painlessly sends 20 watts of power through the skin using the same principle involved in recharging electric toothbrushes.

Impressive as these achievements are, researchers soon became aware that seldom does the entire heart fail. It is far more common for patients to have localised weaknesses or damage. Therefore, in preference to replacing the whole heart, not only a risky, but also an extremely expensive procedure, patients could be treated with a simpler, less invasive device which took over or stimulated the function of part of the heart. These devices are known as "Ventricular Assist Devices" (VADs).

Using such devices, it is often possible for the damaged part of the heart to be "rested" and, after a suitable interval of rest and drug therapy, the patient's heart functions are restored to near normal (1).

6.2.2. Ventricular Assist Devices

Typically the VAD consists of tubes and a pump that effectively reroute blood around the weak or damaged ventricles. There are variants, however, and one such is the intra-aortic balloon pump (IABP). It was introduced by Dr Adrian Kantrowitz in the late 1960s as a simple yet effective device to increase blood flow through the lungs (perfusion). The IABP is a polyethylene balloon mounted on a catheter and filled with helium (easily absorbed into the bloodstream in case of rupture), which is generally inserted into the aorta through the femoral artery in the leg.

The balloon is guided into the descending aorta, and located approximately 2 cm from the left sub-clavian artery. At the beginning of the diastole (the period between two contractions of the heart, when the muscle relaxes and the chamber fills with blood), the balloon inflates, augmenting coronary perfusion.

At the beginning of the systole (the period of the cardiac cycle during which the heart contracts), the balloon deflates, and blood is ejected from the left ventricle. In this way the cardiac output is increased by as much as 40%, the work of the left ventricle is reduced, and the device supports the heart indirectly. The device, which has an on-board battery with power for up to about 2 hours, is programmed and driven by a separate console. Fig. 6.4 shows an IABP device, and its location in the body.

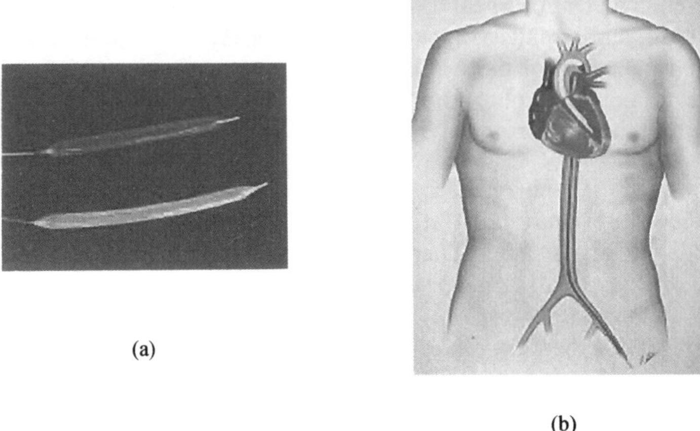

(a)

(b)

Figure 6.4 The intra-aortic balloon pump (IABP) (a) the pump itself (b) the device in situ, (Courtesy the Texas Heart Institute, USA)

Although the IABP worked satisfactorily, medical researchers, led by the redoubtable American heart surgeon Michael DeBakey, were by now convinced that total heart replacement was not necessarily the best treatment for diseased and damaged hearts, were working to develop a range of VADs using different types of blood pump and control systems. Normally the more important of the ventricles is the left one, as it supplies blood to the whole body except the lungs. Therefore the main emphasis was directed towards the perfection of left ventricular assist devices (LVADs), with some attention to stimulation of both ventricles.

Many devices were developed, but essentially only two methods of driving the pump were used: continuous or pulsed, and in the descriptions that follow, I have drawn on an excellent series of research reports produced by the Texas Heart Institute (2).

Continuous Drive Pumping Devices

The refinement of the continuous-flow pump resulted from the chance treatment of a NASA engineer, Jim Akkerman, who pointed out that the way to move large quantities of fluid around small pipes was to use an Archimedes screw. The latest versions of the DeBakey model use a small rotary pump, sewn on to the heart, and driven by a magnetic field, the device being connected to an extra-corporeal controller by a cable.

Other rotary pump VADs include the Jarvik-2000, which fits inside the left ventricle, and receives power either from a fixed jack implanted behind the patient's ear, or via a small cable which exits the body through the abdominal wall. The impellor—the pump's only moving part—is a neodymium-iron-boron magnet, housed inside a welded titanium shell (all the blood-contacting parts are made of highly polished titanium), and runs on ceramic bearings. Another version of the same principle is the Medtronic Bio-Pump, originally developed for cardiopulmonary bypass. The Bio-Pump is an extracorporeal, centrifugal device, capable of providing support for one or both ventricles. The pump consists of an acrylic pump head with inlet and outlet ports at right angles to each other. The impellor, a stack of parallel cones, is driven by an external motor and power console. When the impellor rotates at high speeds, it creates a vortex, which drives the blood through the devices in proportion to the rotational speed. Fig. 6.5 shows the Jarvik 2000 axial flow LVAD

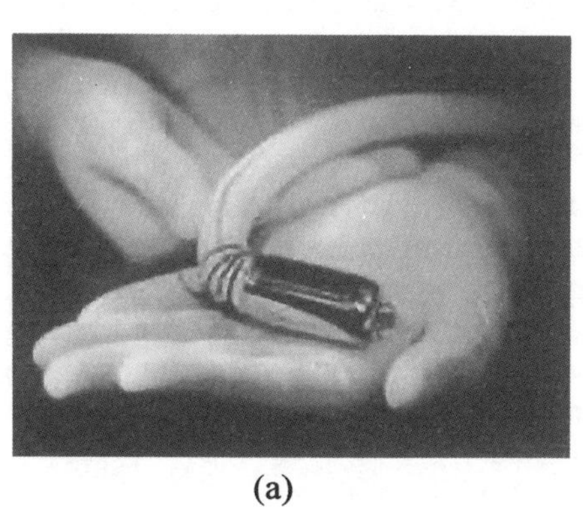

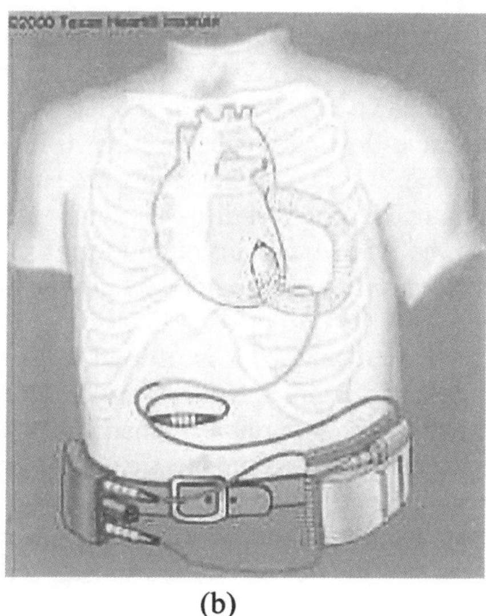

(a)   (b)

Figure 6.5 The Jarvik-2000 LVAD (a) the device itself and (b) the pump in situ (Courtesy the Texas Heart Institute, USA)

Pulsed Drive Pumping Devices

These come in essentially two variants: extra-corporeal and implanted. The first type includes the Abiomed BVS-5000, used for temporary left, right, or biventricular support. It was the first (1988) heart assist device approved by the FDA for the support of post-cardiotomy patients (those who have developed heart failure as a result of heart surgery). The system is similar to the natural heart in having two chambers; in this case made from polyurethane. The atrial chamber is filled with blood by gravity, and then is vented outside the patient. The ventricular chamber is connected to the power source by an air line; the atrial and ventricular chamber are separated by two tri-leaflet valves.

The Thoratec Ventricular Assist Device again can provide left, right, or biventricular support. The blood pump, contained in a rigid plastic case with a flexible (polyurethane) pumping sac, is connected to tubes inserted into the heart. The drive console delivers air to the blood pump in a pulse-like fashion, causing blood to be expelled into the aorta and/or pulmonary artery. Three different modes of operation are available: asynchronous (pumping occurs at a preset rate), synchronous (pumping is synchronised with the patient's heart rate), or volume mode (pumping is adjusted according to the left ventricular capacity).

Implantable pulsed devices include; the Model-7 Abdominal Left Ventricular Assist Device (ALVAD, a pneumatic single chambered pump, which is placed in the abdomen and connected to the left ventricle by a Dacron tube. Blood from the left ventricle flows through the tube, filling a polyurethane sac contained in a titanium housing. Air is introduced into the space between the sac and the housing, and blood is pumped through a disc-valve into the aorta. With the exception of the valve discs, and the inflow and outflow port grafts, all blood-contacting surfaces are coated with polyester fibres to promote the growth of a cellular lining.

A similar system is offered by the HeartMate, a device also implanted in the abdominal cavity. Noteworthy features are the use of porcine valves in the two circuits, and a portable rechargeable battery pack, worn around the waist, which gives the patient complete freedom of movement for up to 8 hours. An interesting advance, operated by remote control, is the Penn State Lionheart, an implantable assist pump with no wires passing through the skin. The device comprises a small sac which inflates and deflates inside a rigid casing.

All the experience gained so far with LVADs is that patients enjoy a high quality of life while awaiting transplantation, and there are even unexpected benefits.. Transplant centres have frequently noticed that patients awaiting a donor heart, and using LVADs, were recovering. The total rest to the left ventricle afforded by the device was reversing the heart failure, and the enlarged cells in the left ventricle were returning to their normal size, whenever the heart degeneration was spotted early enough. Fig. 6.6 shows three examples of pulsed VADs, which use a considerable variety of different materials and fabrication techniques to achieve biocompatibility.

External Blood Pump

(a)

Battery
Pack and
Computer
Controller
Blood Pump
Implanted in
the Chest
Cavity
Power Cord
Protruding
through the
Skin

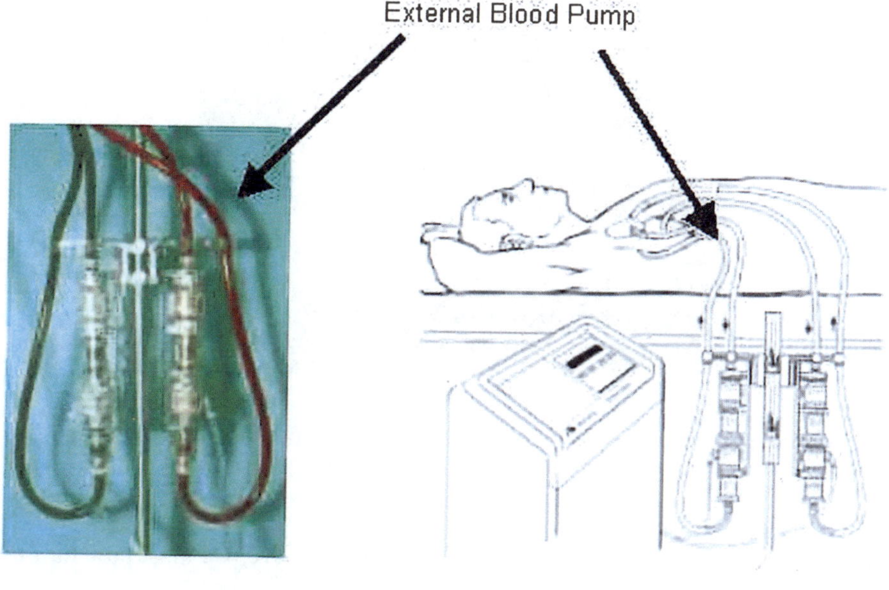

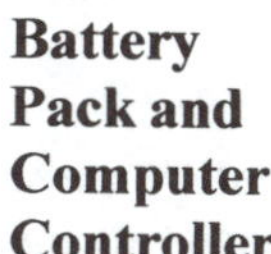

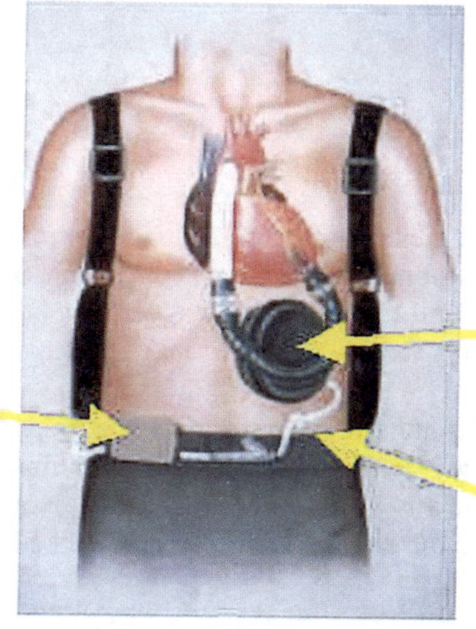

(b)

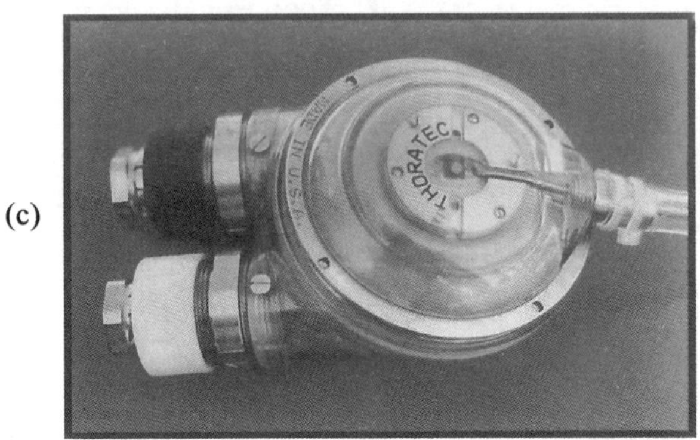

Figure 6.6 Three pulsed ventricular assist devices (a) the Abiomed BVS-5000 (b) the HeartMate (c) the Thoratec VAD (Courtesy the Texas Heart Institute, USA)

From the series of active implants we have considered above, we must now turn to those which are used to promote healing, but do so in a passive way.

6.3. Holding Things Together

6.3.1. Sutures

Non-Absorbable Sutures

Sutures have been used as a means of closing wounds for many centuries: the earliest recorded use of gut sutures being by the Greek physician Galen in 175 AD. Since then, over the centuries, natural materials, such as leather, horse hair, flax, cotton and silk have all been successfully used.

The development of synthetic polymers in the mid 20th century gave the surgeon nylon and polyester, and the choice was then further widened to include polyethylene, polypropylene and other textile materials. Nowadays sutures are often supplied already attached to the needle, sterilised and packed ready for use in plastic containers.

In order to perform satisfactorily sutures have to satisfy a number of property requirements, which include:

   *   Physical

* Handling
* Biological

Whilst the nature of the material (Chapter 2) will have a lot to do in the feel and handling of the suture, the make up of the sutures themselves is also important. For example, although monofilament sutures are generally easy to use, and offer little resistance to passage through tissue, they may not provide a secure knot. Braided sutures, on the other hand, are—for the same overall diameter—more flexible, and the knots tend to be more secure. The application of a coating to braided sutures, also achieves two objecives: they are easier to use, and the smooth surface prevents the entrapment of bacteria.

The type of suture I have just described, whether made from natural or synthetic polymers, or even metals, being non-absorbable—in that they are not absorbed by the body—usually have to be removed after the wound has healed.

Absorbable (Resorbable) Sutures

A second category comprises absorbable sutures, also made from natural or synthetic polymer, but absorbed by the body. There are two main advantages of using absorbable sutures:

* Less likelihood of infection
* Lower chance of provoking a damaging immune reaction.

By their very nature this type of suture tends to lose most of its tensile strength in less than 60 days, which is more than sufficient for most purposes.

It is convenient to divide absorbable sutures into two types: natural and synthetic. The natural variety are prepared from the mucosa (mucous membrane) or submucosa (the layer of loose connective tissue underlying the mucosa) of sheep or beef intestines, and they are broken down—as is gut, which comes from beef intestine—by enzymatic degradation.

Synthetic sutures are mainly found in four categories: polyglactin, polyglycolic acid, polydioxanone, and polyglecaprone (3). These materials are designed to interact with water and break down into smaller units, which are then consumed by macrophages (the large scavenger cells present in major organs and many types of tissue), and the residues excreted as carbon dioxide and water (4). A number of factors, which can be used to create specific properties, affect the rate of degradation, including the size and shape of the molecule, its crystallinity, and the length of the polymer chain (molecular weight).

Generally, crystalline structures, such as the homopolymers polydioxanone are more resistant to degradation than the largely amorphous copolymers polyglactin and polyglycolic acid, since it is more difficult for the water molecules to penetrate the denser crystalline regions. Molecules with longer polymer chains (see Chapter 2) are also more resistant.

To make them more acceptable, and to control the rate of absorption, gut sutures have also been coated with a biocompatible and biodegradable polyurethane. The incorporation of chromium into the tanning process of the gut is also found to increases absorption time. The repeat units in the polymer chains of the four polymers discussed above are shown below in Fig. 6.7.

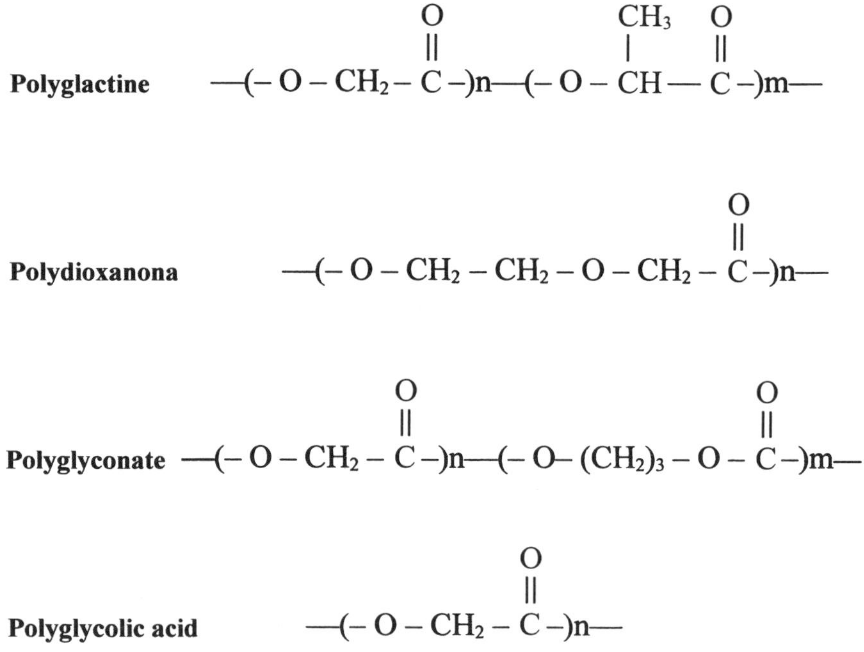

$$\textbf{Polyglactine} \quad -\!\!\!\left(-O-CH_2-\overset{\overset{\displaystyle O}{\|}}{C}-\right)\!n\!-\!\!\!\left(-O-\overset{\overset{\displaystyle CH_3}{|}}{CH}-\overset{\overset{\displaystyle O}{\|}}{C}-\right)\!m\!-$$

$$\textbf{Polydioxanona} \quad -\!\!\!\left(-O-CH_2-CH_2-O-CH_2-\overset{\overset{\displaystyle O}{\|}}{C}-\right)\!n\!-$$

$$\textbf{Polyglyconate} \quad -\!\!\!\left(-O-CH_2-\overset{\overset{\displaystyle O}{\|}}{C}-\right)\!n\!-\!\!\!\left(-O-(CH_2)_3-O-\overset{\overset{\displaystyle O}{\|}}{C}-\right)\!m\!-$$

$$\textbf{Polyglycolic acid} \quad -\!\!\!\left(-O-CH_2-\overset{\overset{\displaystyle O}{\|}}{C}-\right)\!n\!-$$

Figure 6.7 Chemical structures of the repeat chain units of four types of absorbable suture materials

6.3.2. *Resorbable Wound Healing Devices*

Normally, the peritoneum (the lining of the abdomen and the organs located within it), which is composed of an outer, continuous, layer of mesothelial cells, starts to repair any damage within 48 hours, and usually the process is complete within 7 days.

One of the most significant complications which can follow general abdominal, gynaecological, orthopaedic and cardiac surgery, is the formation of adhesions (the union of two normally separate surfaces). These can have potentially serious clinical consequences, including bowel obstruction, abdominal and pelvic pain, infertility, and problems with subsequent operations on the same site.

The most powerful causes of adhesion formation are peritoneal trauma (in this case trauma simply means a wound) and ischaemia (restricted blood supply), although it can be caused by foreign bodies; often containing silica, such as talc, starch from surgical gloves and lint from surgical gauze.

The mechanism of adhesion formation is complex, and involves the interaction of many different cell types. In simple terms, any damage to the peritoneum releases a fibrin-rich exudate (see Chapter 3) capable of inducing adhesion in as little as 3 hours. The normal agent for promoting such a process is tPA (tissue plasminogen activator), whose activity is decreased following surgery. After 5 days the adhesion has become organised into a fibrous network, and begins to develop its own blood supply. Various attempts have been made to prevent, or minimise, adhesions, including modified surgical techniques, and drug therapy, without any marked success. The most important, however, are to minimise trauma-induced damage, and the elimination of sources of infection. An encouraging technique is to separate the two surfaces until healing has taken place. The requirements of such a physical barrier are as follows:

* Persists during critical stages of healing
* No effect on healing process
* Bioresorbable
* Does not promote bacterial growth
* Easy to use

Most types of natural barriers have, not surprisingly, tended to promote adhesion instead of preventing it, and a range of synthetic materials has been tried, including the following:

* Oxidised regenerated cellulose – fairly successful
* Expanded polytetrafluorethylene (PTFE) – good but non-resorbable
* Liquid barriers – mixed success, rapidly dispersed and absorbed

More encouraging results have been made with polymeric membranes based on hyaluronic acid (HA), either alone, or in combination with carboxymethylcellulose

(CMC). This type of material is manufactured by the Genzyme Corporation in the US and UK, and marketed under the name Seprafilm™. The membrane is applied after surgery, and before closure, and adheres well to moist tissue. It turns to a gel in approximately 24–48 hours, but is capable of keeping the two surfaces apart for up to 7 days. It is cleared from the body within 28 days.

The use of such barrier membranes is, of course, more necessary—and easier—where open surgery is used. Microsurgical and minimally invasive surgical procedures may not, in all cases require such separation, but—when they do—the procedures become rather more complicated.

6.4. Limb Extension Techniques

6.4.1. Traction

We saw in Chapter 4 how materials are used in a variety of applications and combinations to support parts of the body, either to promote healing of a fracture or strain, or to correct a misalignment. Now we should consider the use of a pulling force, traction, to treat muscle and skeleton disorders. Traction is usually applied to the arms and legs, the neck, backbone, or the pelvis. It is used to treat fractures, dislocations, and long-duration muscle spasms, and also to prevent or correct deformities. There are two main types of traction:

* Skin traction
* Skeletal traction

In the former, weights are attached either through adhesive, or non-adhesive tape, boots or cuffs; while the latter is chosen when more pulling force is needed than can be withstood by skin traction, or when the part of the body needing traction is positioned so that skin traction is impossible. A case where skin traction would not be appropriate is when it is necessary to produce a twisting motion of, say, the pelvis.

Skeletal traction requires the placement of tongs, pins or screws into the bones so that the force is applied directly to the bone. The placement and removal is generally done under general anaesthetic. In minor case, however, a local anaesthetic may be sufficient. Since they are not intended to remain in the body for very protracted periods, the implanted components are usually made from stainless steel. It is, however, necessary to maintain a high standard of cleanluness so as to minimise the risk of infection.

Fig. 6.8 Illustrates several different forms of both skin and skeletal traction.

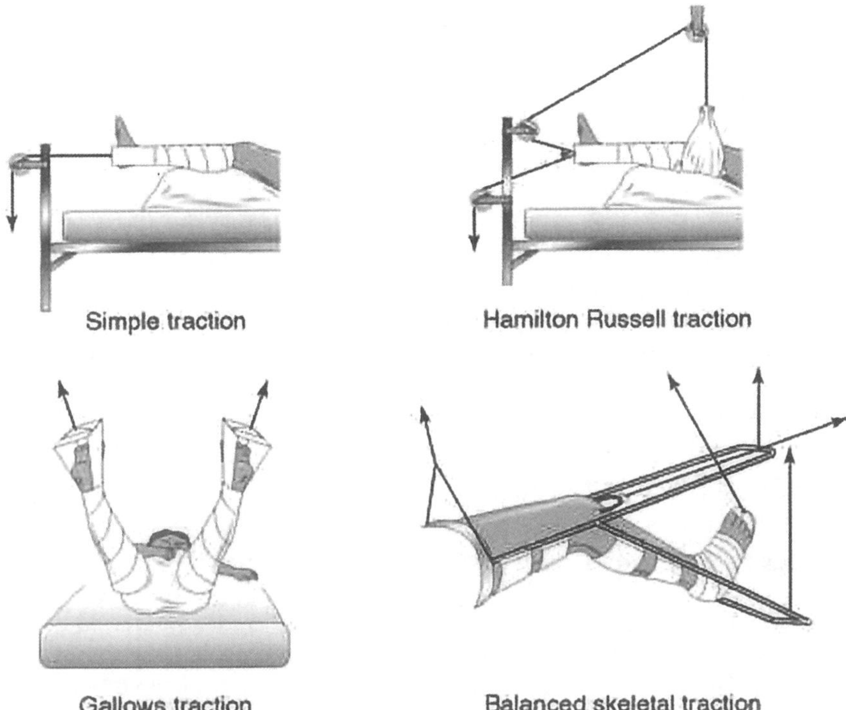

Figure 6.8 Different forms of skin and skeletal traction (Courtesy the Dr Joseph F Smith Medical Library, Wausau, USA)

Alternatively, it may be necessary to induce a degree of flexion into a joint, such as the elbow or wrist. A novel device, produced by Thera Tech Equipment Inc., USA, (Fig. 6.9) provides the necessary tension.

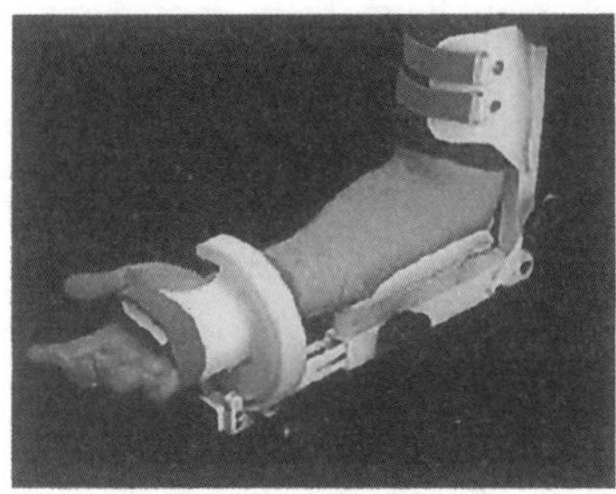
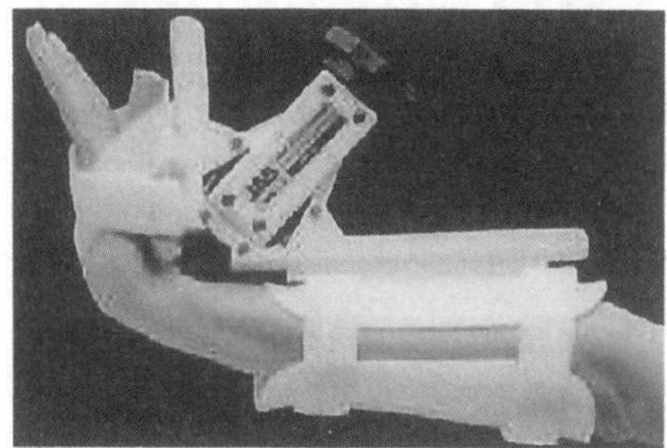

Figure 6.9 Examples of the JAS Progressive Stretch Splints (Courtesy Thora Tech Equiupment Inc.)

6.4.2. Extension

On occasions where it is necessary to apply continuous extension to a limb, perhaps after an operation to treat a shortened leg, the process is applied very slowly, so as to allow the growth of new bone.

Here pins are inserted into the bone on either side of the fracture, and connected to a collar. The two collars are joined by screwed rods, and extension is achieved by tightening nuts placed on the rods, by a predetermined amount every day or week. Again the implanted components and rods are made of stainless steel, with some of the ancillary parts made from nylon.

It is worth recalling the adjustable frame used in neurosurgery to immobilise the head (Chapter 1), although in that case the purpose was positioning rather than extension.

6.5. Pins, Patches and Plates

In addition to the applications already discussed, there are many occasions in which it is appropriate to implant materials into the body to provide temporary support or protection. These include pins and plates to hold parts of a fractured bone together, the use of metal staples in certain types of wound repair, and the use of metal patches to cover holes or gaps in the skull.   Because of its good biocompatibility stainless steel or titanium are the most favoured candidates.

Interestingly enough, although we are here considering short or medium term implantation, there are cases where people have carried around pieces of metal in their bodies for many decades with no apparent inconvenience. Most noteworthy are the fragments of shrapnel resulting from gunshot wounds, which are certainly neither clean nor biocompatible! The mechanism for this is not entirely clear, but it seems likely that the acceptability of such inclusions may have been increased by the development of an oxide film on the surface, or even that the metal is located in a region where there is little blood flow, and the immune system has been fooled into ignoring the intruder! More likely, though, is that the implant has encouraged the production of a capsule of fibrous tissue, which insulates the foreign body from the patrolling cells.

6.6. Conclusion

As can be appreciated, the question of whether or not an implant can be considered to be temporary or permanent depends on a variety of circumstances, including the effect of the body on the implant, and vice versa, as well as the healing characteristics of the condition..

It is appropriate now to turn to the class of implant which I have deemed to be permanent, and which I have subdivided into two categories: load-bearing and non-load bearing. Both demand similar high standards of biocompatibility and chemical resistance, but the former—in some applications which may involve strong physical exercise—need to withstand forces exceeding the weight of the body, accompanied by severe torsional stresses.

References

(1) Sternberg S., 'Artificial Hearts Pumping Ahead,' USA Today, October (2000)
(2) Texas Heart Institute, 'Leading Wit the Heart,' 1996-2000
(3) 'Sutures' http:/www.sas.upenn.sdu/-kbader/sutures.htm
(4) 'Influence of soluble suture factors on in vitro macrophage function', Uff Biomaterials, 16 (1995) 355-360

Chapter 7

Permanent Implants

7.1. Introduction

So far we have considered materials and devices which are in the main passively implanted in the body for relatively short periods. Now we must turn to another group of implants, such as: mechanical heart valves, as well as complex machinery, eg pacemakers, artificial hearts and other cardiac assist devices, cosmetic, and oral implants. Whilst both have to withstand the effects of rejection and the action of the body fluids, the former have also to operate mechanically over long periods of time.

7.2. Artificial Heart Valves

We saw in Chapter 1 that the heart is essentially a pump, whose function is to deliver oxygen-rich blood to the arteries, and thence to the cells, so that they may receive the oxygen necessary for their survival. The blood flow is controlled by the heart valves, and Fig. 1.7 shows the arrangement of the valves within the heart itself. Fig. 7.1 depicts a section through the heart showing the location of the four valves.

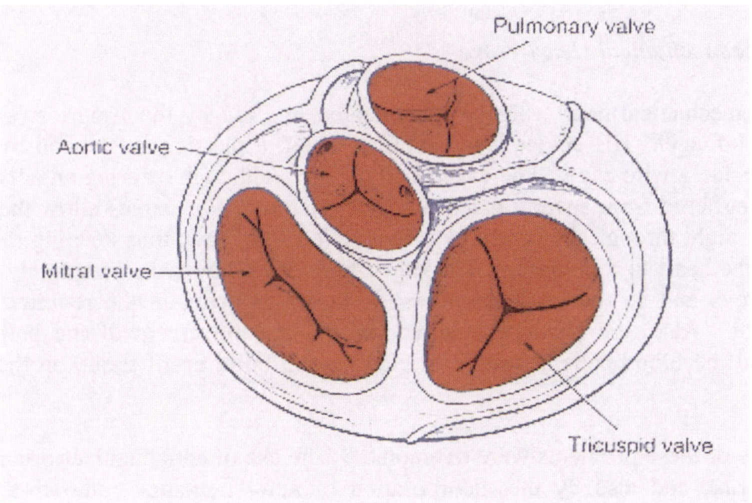

Figure 7.1 The layout of the four valves in the heart

Once the blood has given up its oxygen, it enters the right atrium, which then contracts, forcing the blood down through the tricuspid valve into the right ventricle.

125

This chamber then contracts, pushing the blood through the pulmonary valve to receive its supply of oxygen. This completed, the enriched blood returns to the left atrium, from which it passes through the mitral valve into the left ventricle. From the left ventricle the blood passes through the aortic valve into the aorta, which distributes it to the rest of the body.

Although there are many different diseases of the heart valves, they fall into two main categories:

* Stenosis
* Incompetence

The stenotic heart valve prevents the valve from opening fully due to stiffening of the valve tissue, thus requiring more work to push the blood through the valve. Incompetent heart valves permit backflow of the blood, and thus cause too little blood to circulate round the body.

Should it become necessary to replace one or more of the heart valves, the surgeon has two different alternatives: either to use a mechanical heart valve or a tissue valve.

7.2.1. The Mechanical Heart Valve

The first mechanical heart valve was implanted in 1952 by the American surgeon Charles Hufnagel. His device was simplicity itself, a plastic tube topped by a ball located inside a wire cage. The caged-ball concept, although offering an acceptable solution, suffered from several disadvantages. Natural heart valves allow the blood to flow straight through the centre of the valve (central flow), thus keeping the work done by the heart to a minimum. The caged-ball valve, however, completely blocks central flow, and so the heart has to work harder to maintain the required blood throughput. Also, the changes in direction and the movement of the ball cause damage to the blood cells, resulting in clotting and build up of tissue on the valve seating.

Some of these problems were overcome by the use of anticoagulant drugs (such as Warfarin), and also by the incorporation of new "non-stick" smooth-surfaced materials, eg Teflon (PTFE or polytetrafluorethylene) and Mylar (polyethylene terephthalate) into the construction of the valve, and thus to offer less frictional resistance to the blood flow. Early in the 1960s, a surgeon Albert Starr and a retired engineer Lowell Edwards, further improved the design by using a metal ball instead of a plastic one; and giving the seating a sharp edge. This served to provide a chopping motion when the ball moved, so that any invasive tissue was cut away as fast as it formed.

Although Starr-Edwards valves are still in use today, the mid 1960s saw the introduction of a new concept: the tilting-disk valve. This type of valve has a polymer disk held in place by two welded struts. The disk floats between the two struts in such a way as to close when the blood begins to flow backwards, and re-opens when the flow is reversed. This design was found to be vastly superior to the caged-ball model, in providing central flow while at the same time preventing backflow.

Fig. 7.2 Shows examples of these two types of mechanical heart valves; and how the former was stitched into place.

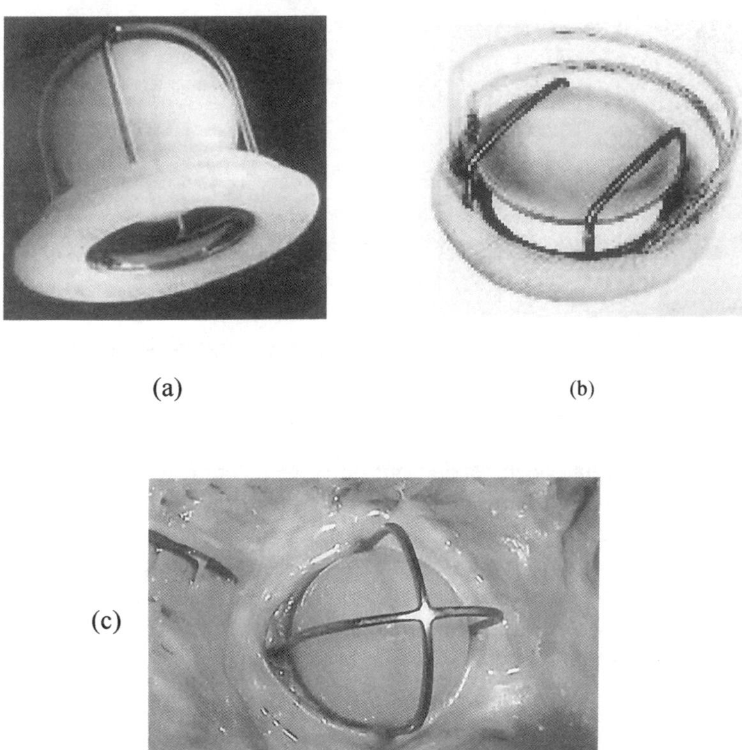

(a) (b)

(c)

Figure 7.2 Mechanical heart valves (a) a caged ball valve (b) the tilting-disk valve (c) the former in position

Many manufacturers throughout the world now offer tilting-disk valves, each with its own claimed advantages, and much research work has centred on improvements in flow-path design. These include increasing the opening angle from the original 60^0 to 70^0; strengthening the outlet struts, and the use of more advanced materials.

In 1979 a new design of mechanical heart valve was introduced, the "bileaflet" valve, comprising two semi-circular leaflets which pivot on hinges. The leaflets, made of pyrolytic carbon, swing open parallel to the blood flow. With certain designs the leaflets do not close completely, allowing a small amount of backflow. Nevertheless, this concept is the one most widely used, with a US market share of over 90%. The Medtronic-Hall valve leads the tilting-disk field, and the St. Jude valve is foremost among the bileaflet candidates. Fig. 7.3 shows both types of valve.

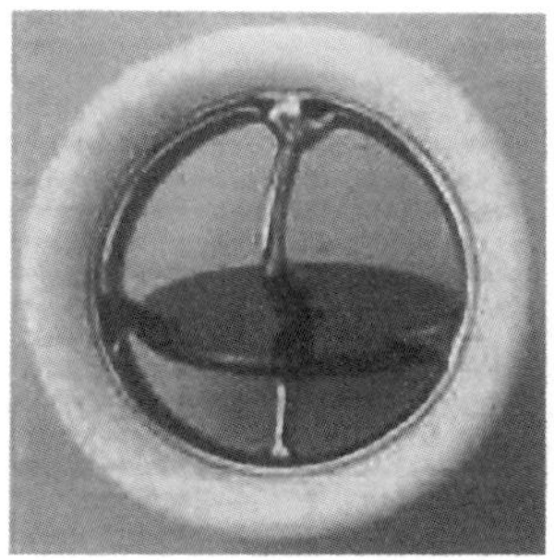 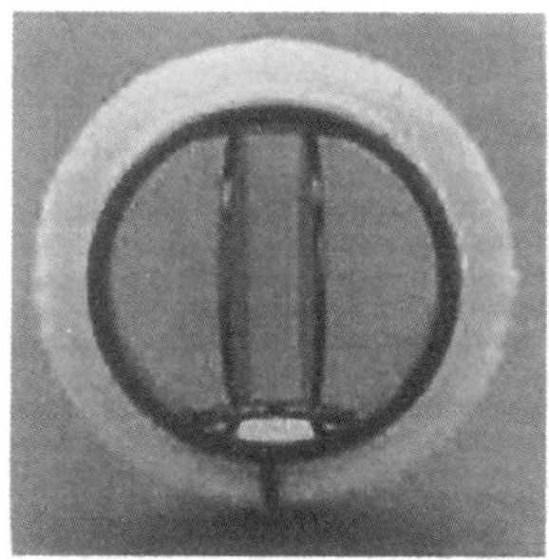

(a)   (b)

Figure 7.3 Two modern mechanical heart valves (a) The Medtronic Hall Tilting-Disk Valve (b) the St. Jude Medical Hinged Bileaflet Prosthesis.

As always much effort has been carried out on ways to improve the performance of mechanical heart valves. The quest has been for better flow design, and components which combine mechanical tolerance to repeated movement, as well as materials which do not cause clotting in the blood stream. The most commonly used materials are stainless steel alloys, molybdenum alloys, tungsten, titanium, pyrolytic carbon and pyrolytic carbon coated graphite; silicone rubbers, PTFE, and polyester fabric for the sewing rings; which allow the valve to be stitched in place.

7.2.2. Tissue Valves

An alternative to the use of mechanical heart valves is provided by prosthetic tissue valves, of which there are essentially two types: human tissue valves and animal tissue valves. Both types are also known as bioprosthetic valves, and they offer several advantages over mechanical valves. Firstly their design can more closely approximate to the natural human valve. Secondly, they do not require long-term anticoagulants. Thirdly, they have better haemodynamics (bloodflow capacity) and so do not cause damage to blood cells. Finally, they do not suffer from many of the structural problems experienced by mechanical valves.

Where human tissue valves are used, the techniques employed often differ, depending upon whether the replacement valve (graft) comes from another person (homograft), or from the same patient into which it is implanted (autograft). In the former case, the procedure is similar in many ways to that described in Chapter 1 for kidney transplantation. The recipient is likely to suffer minimal rejection problems, and will not require any immunosuppressive therapy.

In the case of autografts, the most common method is the Ross procedure, which is used for the replacement of diseased aortic valves. The aortic valve is removed, and the patient's pulmonic valve is transplanted to the aortic position. The pulmonic valve is then generally replaced by a homograft. The Ross procedure requires a considerable amount of surgical skill to tailor the incoming valves to their new sites. The advantage is that the patient receives a living valve in the aortic position, which offers a greater chance of long term survival than any other type of valve replacement.

After 20 years only 15% of patients need additional work, and—where a pulmonary artery homograft has been used to replace the pulmonary valve—the success rate in the USA is reported to be 94% after 5 years and 83% after 20 years.

As an alternative to the use of human tissue, we can use animal tissue (a hetero- or xenograft), the most commonly employed being porcine (valve tissue from a pig), and bovine pericardial tissue (from a cow). The leaflet tissues are generally stiffened by a tanning solution, such as glutaraldehyde.

Several different procedures are available for the implantation of animal tissue valves. The most familiar method is for the leaflets to be sewn to a metal wire former (stent) bent to form three U-shaped prongs. A polyester sewing skirt is attached to the rim of the stent, and the stent itself is covered with polyester cloth. The procedure is the same for both porcine and bovine tissue, except that—in the latter case—the small metal cylinder which joins together the ends of the stent, is located in the middle of one of the post loops. Inevitably, the use of a stent in which the leaflets are sewn inside the ring, will reduce the size of the usual opening. This can be overcome by the use of a "stentless" valve, which is made by removing the entire aortic root and adjacent block, which is then trimmed and implanted into the patient. Fig. 7.4 shows some types of animal tissue valves currently available to the surgeon.

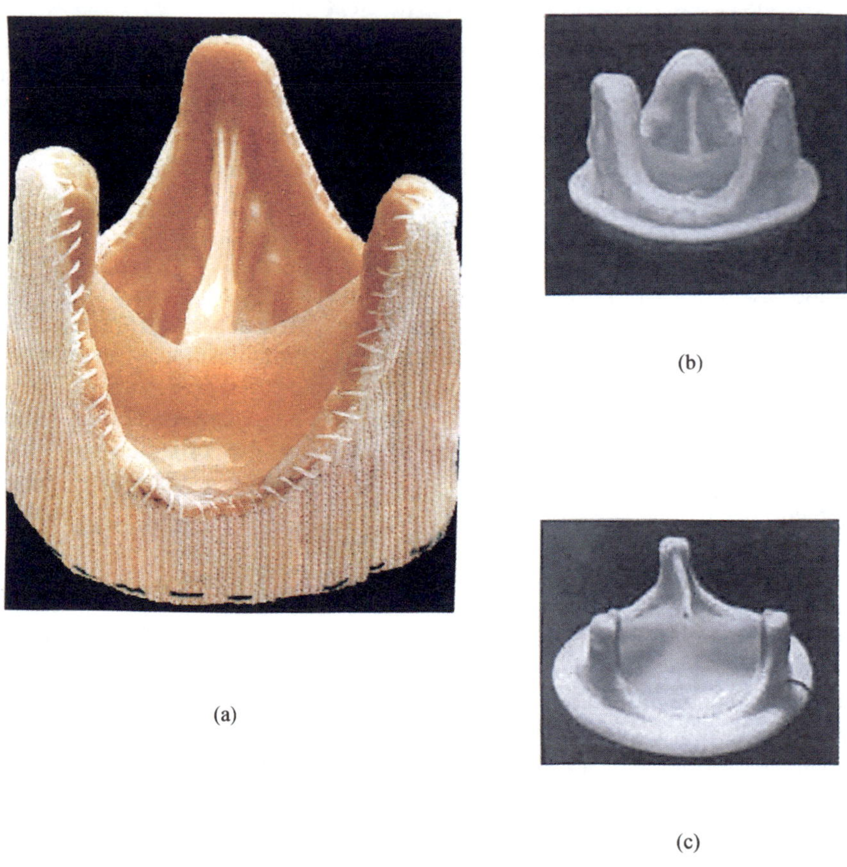

(a)

(b)

(c)

Figure 7.4 Some examples of animal tissue valves (a) a bioprosthetic valve made from natural heart tissue mounted on a polymer scaffold (b) a bovine pericardial valve (c) a stentless porcine valve

Another variation uses a single piece of bovine pericardium mounted on the outside of the stent, instead of being sewn to the inner edge. The manufacturers claim that such a valve with a 19 mm opening gives the same flow characteristics as a 23 mm porcine stented valve (1), almost the full size of that in a healthy heart. The stent is made from acetal homopolymer, because of its high dimensional stability, and the sewing ring is made from a medical grade of silicone.

Whilst clearly both mechanical and tissue valves are, quite literally, life-saving prostheses they do suffer from a number of disadvantages, some of them serious. Mechanical valves are very durable, although a recent analysis (2) has shown that some pyrolytic carbon leaflets have been found to suffer from fatigue. The barely audible click of the opening and shutting sequence can be distasteful to some wearers. However, the main disadvantage is the tendency to produce clotting.

Bioprosthetic valves, while free from the clotting problem, are less durable and have to be replaced more frequently. A study undertaken by the University of Southern California School of Medicine (3) has shown that for the first 10 years of use, there is no difference in mortality rates between valve types, but that after 10 years the rate is higher for those with a bioprosthetic valve. However, the difference is seen only in patients who received the replacement valves when aged under 65. The inference appears to be that younger patients should receive a mechanical valve in preference to a bioprosthetic one.

A promising solution seems to be offered by the technique of tissue engineering, whereby heart valves have been "grown" in the laboratory from animal cells. We shall consider this, and other bioengineering procedures, in Chapter 10.

7.3. Cardiac Assist Devices — Pacemakers

In order to fulfil its function of collecting and pumping the blood throughout the body, the heart depends on tiny electrical impulses which are passed from the upper to the lower chambers.

These impulses usually start at the heart's natural pacemaker (the sinu-atrial (SA)) node; which is a microscopic area of specialised cardiac muscle situated in the upper wall of the right atrium, causing the atrial muscles to contract. Each impulse travels from the upper chambers into the lower ones via the atrioventricular (AV) node. The impulses pass along a system of fibres, which fan out through the muscles of the ventricle, causing them to contract. This contraction is what we know as a heartbeat. The SA node normally operates at about 100 beats per minute, which is throttled back to 60–80 times per minute by the body's parasympathetic nervous system, which is controlled by the brain. Different reasons, such as disease or age-related processes can disturb the natural heart rhythm.

Two of the most common are:

* A malfunction of the sinus node, (known as sick sinus syndrome), in which the impulses are generated irregularly, or too slowly

                    Life-enhancing Plastics

    * The AV block, where the electrical conduction paths between the atrium and ventricle are interrupted.

In either case, the heart can be assisted through the use of an artificial pacemaker. Fig. 7.5 Shows a diagram of the general layout of the heart and the natural pacemaker.

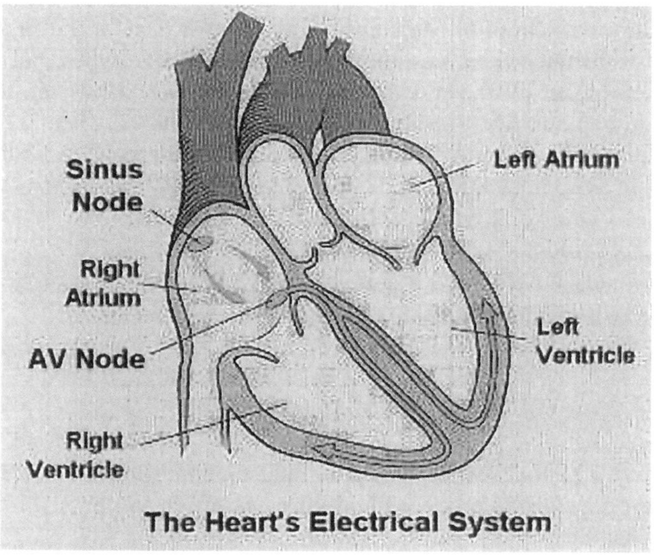

Figure 7.5 The heart showing the components of the natural pacemaker

A mechanical pacemaker is simply a pulse generator complete with battery and lead wire, which transmits electrical signals to the heart muscle. These devices may either be wholly or partially implanted within the body, or—in the case of some more modern adaptations—can perform their function from outside the body. These latter were discussed in Chapter 4.

As in the case of other "active" implants, heart valves, artificial hearts &c., the materials and systems selected have to be acceptable to the body, impervious to its fluids, and capable of operating for long periods with complete reliability. Whilst, as we have seen in Chapter 4, there are pacemakers and other cardiac assist devices that can be worn outside the body, we shall concentrate here on those that are implanted in the body.

The first successful pacemakers were used in the early 1950s, and were connected to the heart by sewing insulated wires (with the ends bared) on to the outside of the heart muscle. This was not altogether successful, since the wires frequently became detached. A better solution was to sew the wire electrodes (loosely folded to absorb the pull of the muscle) directly into the heart muscle. This worked quite well, but the fine wires suffered from fatigue; not surprising since the average heart beats 4×10^7 (40 million) times per year, giving rise to some 80 million flexions. Fig. 7.6 shows one of these early pacemakers, which were contained in an epoxy resin sheath.

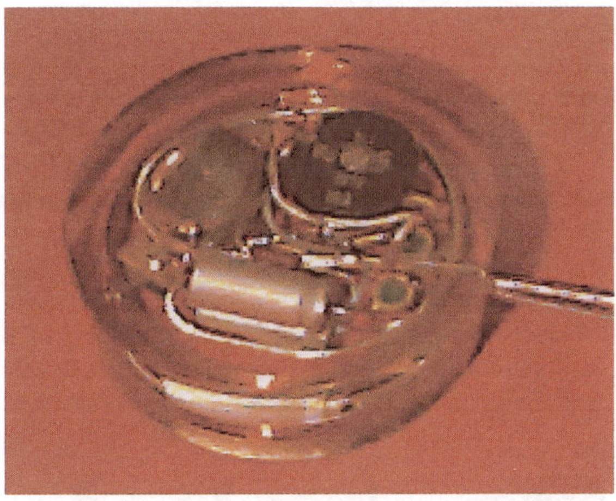

Figure 7.6 A pacemaker from the early 1960s made by Siemens AG, (Courtesy Dr Wolfgang Scheibelhofer, Vienna)

Modern pacemakers are able to sense the heartbeat, and respond accordingly. If it senses that the heartbeat is too slow, or there is no heartbeat, the device emits tiny electrical impulses to pace the heart in order to restore the normal rhythm. When this is achieved, the pacemaker "stands by" until it is needed again.

Depending on the type of therapy required, single or dual-chamber pacemakers are available. In the dual-chamber system, one lead is generally located in the atrium and the other in the ventricle. Many pacemakers are also able to adapt their impulse rate to changing physiological conditions, such as running, gardening, swimming &c., and can contribute the necessary increase in heart rate.

Fig. 7.7 shows the location of a modern dual-chamber pacemaker and the pacing leads.

Dual-chamber pacemaker

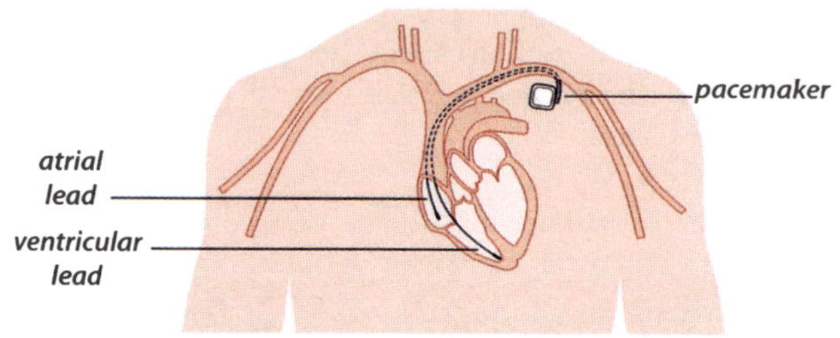

Dual-chamber pacemakers have two leads. One is connected to the right atrium and the other to the right ventricle.

Figure 7.7 A dual-chamber pacemaker in its place (Courtesy British Heart Foundation)

A further refinement in the latest generation of devices, is their capacity to react to mental changes; often accompanied by sudden changes in pulse or blood pressure. This "closed loop" stimulation is a feature of pacemakers made by the German firm Biotronik AG. Fig. 7.8 shows a typical compact modern pacemaker.

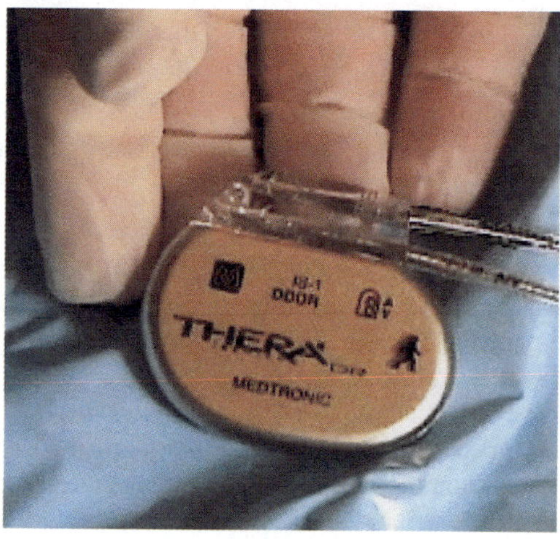

Figure 7.8 A modern pacemaker with titanium casing, (Courtesy Medtronic Inc., USA)

I mentioned earlier the need to have regard to the problems associated with the implantation of "foreign" materials, and this has also been covered at length in Chapter 3. It is now appropriate to consider what materials are available for the construction of the components of cardiac pacemakers and defibrillators. As far as metals are concerned, the most commonly used are titanium, stainless steel, and some of the non-magnetic alloys. This last is becoming more important in view of the increasing exposure of patients to scanning devices (eg MRI &c.).

Polymers are used for cases, some internal components, and to cover the flexible electrical leads. Epoxy and silicone resins are common, but some of the most versatile materials are the polyurethanes. They have good biocompatibility, and—by appropriate choice of the components from which they are made—can be produced in a range of properties; from highly flexible to very rigid. Fig. 7.9 shows the structure of a typical polyurethane molecule, and how it can be modified.

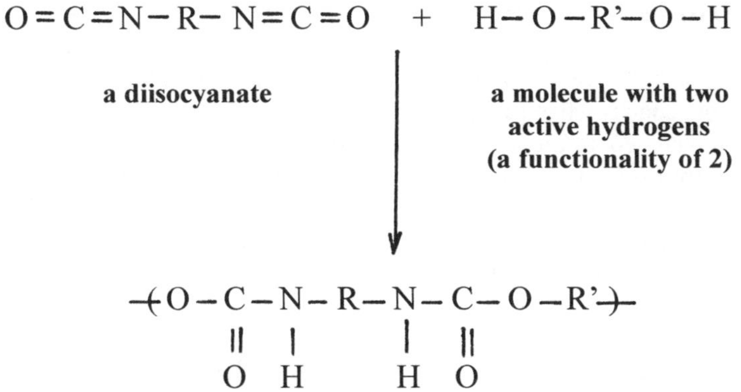

$$O=C=N-R-N=C=O \quad + \quad H-O-R'-O-H$$

a diisocyanate | **a molecule with two active hydrogens (a functionality of 2)**

$$\{O-C-N-R-N-C-O-R'\}$$

a polyurethane

Where R and R' are polymer chains of suiably chosen links

If the active hydrogen-containing molecule has ahigher functionality than 2 (eg 3,4,5,6,7 or 8) increasingly rigid structures will result

Figure 7.9 The structure of a typical polyurethane resin

7.4. Cardiac Assist Devices — Defibrillators

Another condition of the heart which may require electrical intervention is fibrillation, which can be defined as "a rapid and chaotic beating of the many individual muscle fibres of the heart, so that it is consequently unable to maintain the normal, effective pattern of contractions." Fibrillation can take two forms:

* Atrial fibrillation – which results in rapid and irregular heart and pulse rates
* Ventricular fibrillation – where either there is rapid fluctuation of the muscles without any blood being pumped, or the heart stops beating (cardiac arrest).

In its most extreme form, cardiac arrest requires the use of a severe electric shock from externally applied electrodes placed against the chest. Otherwise an internal cardiac defibrillator (ICD) may be used. This is a small lightweight electronic device that is implanted under the skin. It tracks the heart rhythm, and slows down, or halts, excessively rapid heart rates that arise in the ventricles.

The ICD comprises two parts:

* A generator, or tiny computer, with a battery that tracks the heart rhythm, and sends out shocks when required
* A lead attached to the generator, and (preferably) adjacent to the heart so as to monitor the heart rhythm and transmit shocks to the heart.

The operational and construction details are very similar to those already discussed under pacemakers, so I do not propose to go into the matter in more detail here.

So far we have dealt with a range of implants which may be said to have an "active" role. It is now appropriate to turn to another group of materials and prostheses, the long-term "passive" implants, which fall into the general area of cosmetic and reconstructive surgery, in which I have also included dental and maxillo-facial repair work.

7.5. Cosmetic and Reconstructive Surgery

7.5.1. Breast Implants

Of the wide range of different materials used in this application, the overwhelming majority are polymers; and today, most prostheses are made in the form of a thin silicone elastomer capsule with a liquid (generally saline) filling. The simplest form is "round" (or circular), but other variants such as "tear-drop" and specially-designed "custom profiles" are also available. Fig. 7.10 gives examples of the two main forms: round and shaped, together with the necessary dimensions

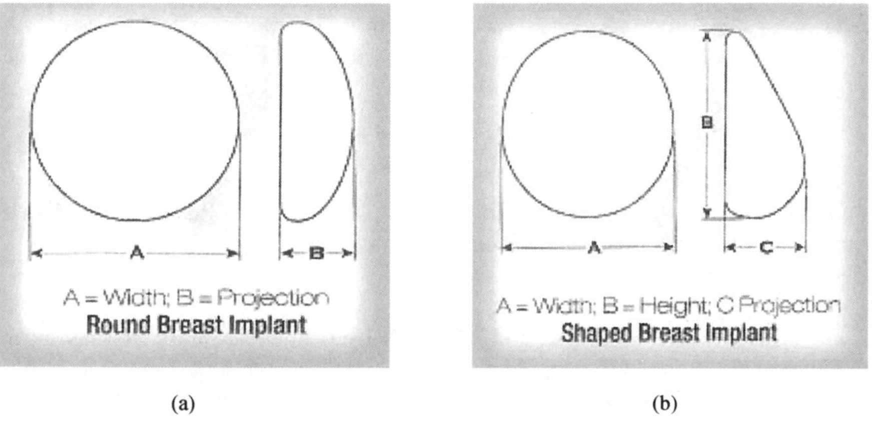

(a)   (b)

Figure 7.10 The two main types of modern breast implants (a) round (b) shaped

In order to understand the reasons for the variety of designs and materials, it is necessary to appreciate why breast implantation is considered necessary, and the relative importance of the different parameters. The first, and oldest, reason is to obtain a more "perfect" figure, either larger or smaller, and the second is for reconstruction purposes, generally following an operation. As in the case of so many medical procedures, breast augmentation was first performed a long time ago. Also, as often happened, the procedures and materials used have been guaranteed, if not to kill, at least to maim!.

Injections of paraffin wax were reported in the 1880s, as was the implantation of glass balls and ivory. The former sometimes caused death by migration to the lung and brain, and the latter must have been extremely uncomfortable. Injections of silicone and other fluids were also tried, but the liquids tended to migrate. This was, to some extent, alleviated by the addition of "fibrosing" agents, such as vegetable oils and fatty acids, but without much success. Silicone products in the form of cross-linked gels were subsequently used, and gave more satisfactory results.

After several years of use in other parts of the body, mainly for rebuilding purposes, plastic implants were used in the form of sponges for augmentation and reconstruction. The materials used included polyethylene, nylon, polyvinyl alcohol (PVA), silicone, PVC and PTFE. Complications soon became apparent, including capsular contracture (an overformation of scar tissue in the normal fibrous capsule that the body forms round the implant), fistulisation (the formation of voids) and infection. Interestingly enough, some work in my own Department at Brunel University showed that pore size in sponges was a critical factor in implantation. Greater than 100 microns (one ten-thousandth of a metre) allowed osteoblasts (bone-forming cells) to enter and start laying down new bone growth. This was ideal to promote the regrowth of fractured or diseased bone, but disastrous for breast implants.

It was not until the early 1960s, when Thomas Cronin and Frank Gerow, in conjunction with the Dow Corning Center for Aid to Medical Research, produced a device consisting of a silicone elastomer capsule filled with silicone gel, that the modern breast implant can be recognised.

The wide diversity of types and materials used in breast implants has largely been dictated by the need to provide a prosthesis which both looks and feels like the real thing, and will keep its shape without deterioration or adverse effects on the body for many years. To that end approval by one of the regulatory bodies, such as the FDA, is essential. The task of providing such an implant is made more difficult, since the human breast has a relatively thin layer of muscle to support it. Many implants were placed under the skin, but outside the pectoral muscles, a procedure that was believed by some to look and feel like an implant. Placing the prosthesis under the muscle layer causes it to be squeezed against the chest, and gives an unnatural look for the first month or so. Later on, however, the muscles act as an internal bra, giving more support and a much more natural look. Fig. 7.11 illustrates the results of this technique.

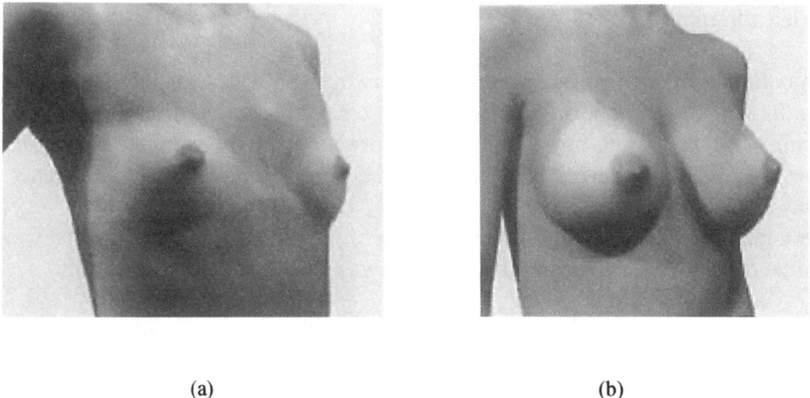

(a) (b)

Figure 7.11 A sub-pectoral breast implant (a) before the operation (b) three months later

The natural look and feel is achieved by careful design of the implant, the materials from which it is made, the substance with which it is filled and how it is distributed inside the shell, by what means it is attached, and also how it is inserted: under the arm, below the breast, at the lower edge of the areola or, very rarely, through the navel. The essential details are briefly summarised as follows.

<u>Design & Composition</u>   Most modern implants comprise a silicone elastomer shell with one, two or three compartments (lumens). These are filled with different liquids according to the desired make-up. Sponge fillings are also used, and—for special applications, for example reconstructions and muscle replacements—solid/foamed silicone elastomers are sometimes implanted.

<u>Shape, Surface & Profile</u>   Shapes vary from round, through oval, contoured (teardrop), crescent, to special custom designed. The shell surface may be plain, textured, or either wholly or partially coated with polyurethane, and the shell material may be one, or several layers (to avoid leakage). The profile (low, moderate or high) is adjusted by the amount of filling to suit the required shape.

<u>Filling & Fixation</u>   One of the major problems with liquid-filled implants has been the possibility of leakage, and the consequent damage to tissue. Accordingly, from the first models—which were filled through a hollow needle, either before or after implantation—many designs of valve have been produced: ranging from simple plug valves, through tubes (which are either tied or plugged), self-seal valves, leaflet valves, to diaphragms. To be successful, the implant must not migrate, and various devices are used to ensure that it stays put. These currently include texturing or profiling the shell surface, and—rather less frequently nowadays—the use of "fixing" tags or patches, often of Dacron (polyester) in the form of loops, mesh patches or felt strips, and polyurethane patches.

<u>Materials</u>   Although several materials have already been mentioned in connection with specific uses, it might be helpful to summarise them here again under their different applications. It should be remembered, however, that not all the materials or materials combinations are still in use; indeed some—eg polyurethane coatings—tend to become detached and broken, and thus may cause damage. There have also been cases of damage, resulting in lawsuits, when liquid silicone has leaked into the breast.

<u>Shells</u>   Silicone elastomer, cured liquid silicone, foamed polyurethane coating adhered by silicone adhesive

<u>Fillings</u>   Silicone, silicone gel, saline solution, dextran, soya oil, polyvinyl pyrrolodone (PVP), also foamed PTFE, polyethylene and polyurethane

<u>Accessories</u> Polyester, polyurethane, varieties of silicone polymers.

To sum up, despite the wide variety of material combinations and the different designs and implantation techniques used over the years, the implants found currently to give the most satisfactory service are made from silicone elastomer and filled either with saline, hydrogel (a mixture of 92% saline and 8% polysaccharides) or, more rarely, silicone gel.

In addition to breast implants for enhancement purposes, where there is no damage to tissue before implantation, we have already seen that there is another category: prostheses used in reconstruction after surgery. A variety of techniques is available, including the use of tissue taken from other areas of the body, such as the abdomen, which may be used alone or in combination with elastomeric silicone implants. Fig. 7.12 illustrates the pre- and post-operativestates of a highly successful breast reconstruction, in which the nipple has also been rebuilt.

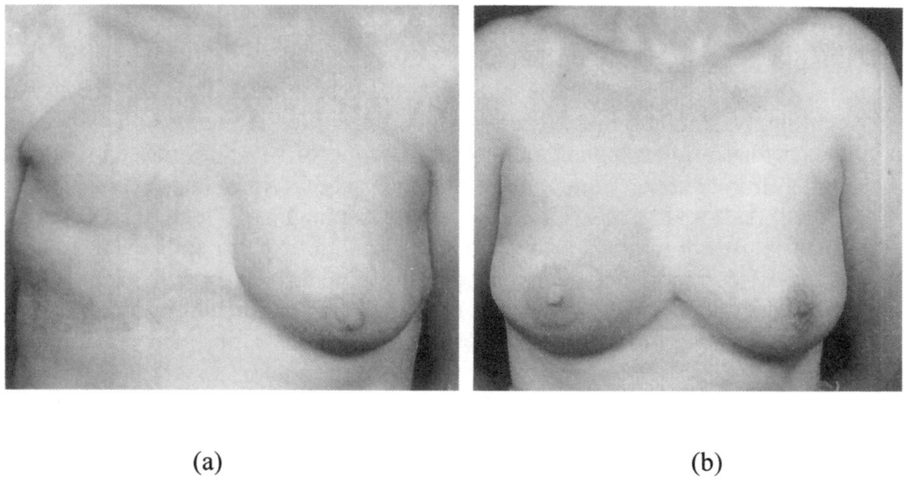

(a)   (b)

Figure 7.12 Breast reconstruction, before and after surgery (Courtesy Mr Michael Brough, The Royal Free Hospital, London)

There is also a wide range of products, either for reconstruction or enhancement, which are worn on the outside of the chest. These are generally made from silicone copolymers, which are lighter than the homopolymer, and—as they are individually crafted—can be made virtually indistinguishable from the natural breast. They may either be worn separately in the bra, or adhered to the skin by means of a flexible adhesive. Fig. 7.13 shows an example of the latter type.

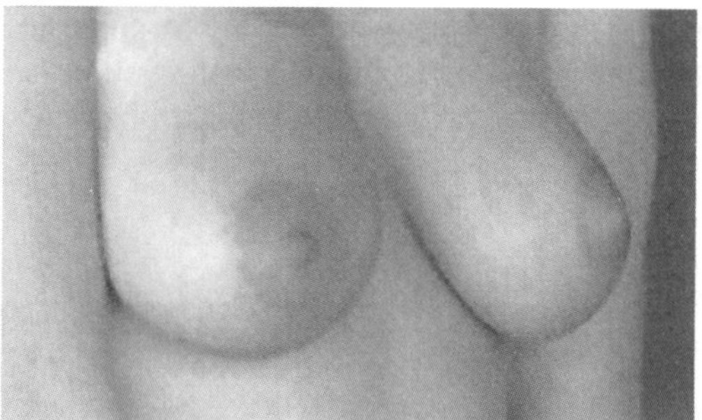

Figure 7.13 A silicone–siloxane breast form

7.5.2. Implantation into Other Areas

Natural tissue or plastics implants are used for enhancement or reconstruction of the pectoral muscles, calves, cheeks and also the chin. Fig. 7.14 shows a dramatic and highly successful repair of the lower part of the face, where the jaw has been reconstruted with part of the fibula. Some of the newer techniques, including the development and use of "artificial" muscles are considered in Chapter 10.

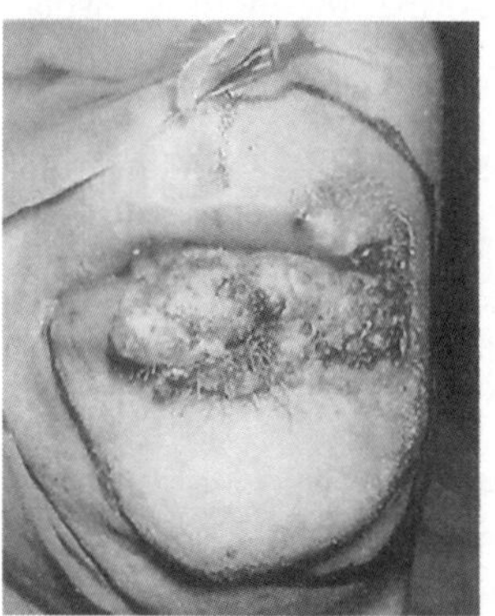
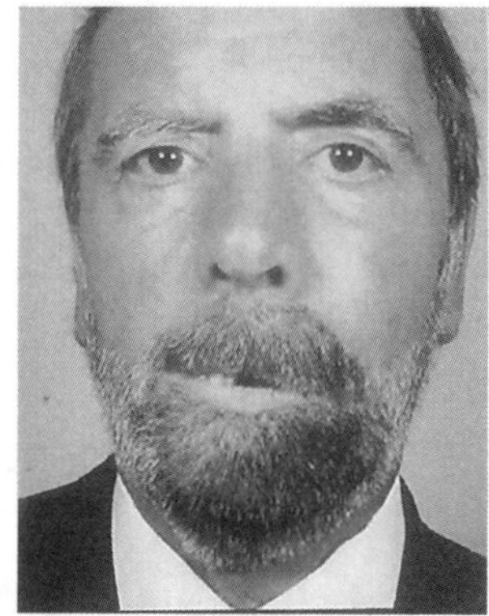

Figure 7.14 Reconstruction of the lower part of the face following cancer of both lips (Courtesy Mr Michael Brough, The Royal Free Hospital, London)

7.6. Dental and Other Facial Implants

Although dentistry is an important independent discipline, it is closely allied to medicine, so it is appropriate to consider its procedures here. Perhaps even more importantly, though, dentistry is a field in which all the classes of materials—metals, plastics, and ceramics—are used for a wide variety of purposes. It will be possible only to give a brief summary of the techniques employed in dentistry, and—for the purposes of this book—it is convenient to divide the subject into two categories:

* General Dentistry
* Reconstructive Surgery of the Jaw

7.6.1. *General Dentistry*

Whilst the baby teeth are important in guiding the growth of the jaw, and the positioning of the permanent (adult) teeth, it is the latter with which we are concerned. The adult tooth is essentially formed from a bone-like material called dentin(e), and comprises two components: the crown and the root, the latter being embedded in a socket in the jaw. The outer surface of the crown is covered by a protective enamel (the hardest substance in the human body).

Inside the crown and root is the pulp, which contains the nerves, connective tissue, blood vessels and lymphatics. The root itself is covered by a bony material called the cementum, which anchors supporting fibres to the tooth. The other ends of the fibres are secured to the bone of the jaw, so that the tooth is suspended in a "hammock-like" structure.

Adults normally have 32 permanent teeth, of which 4 (molars) are commonly called the "wisdom" teeth). Fig. 7.15 shows a cross-section through a tooth, and also the arrangement of the teeth in the mouth.

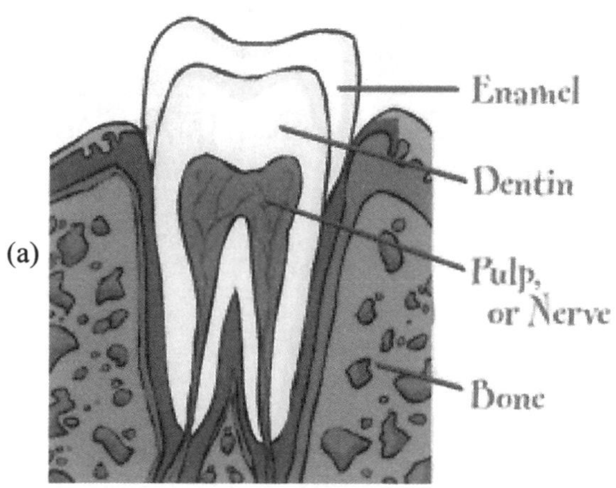

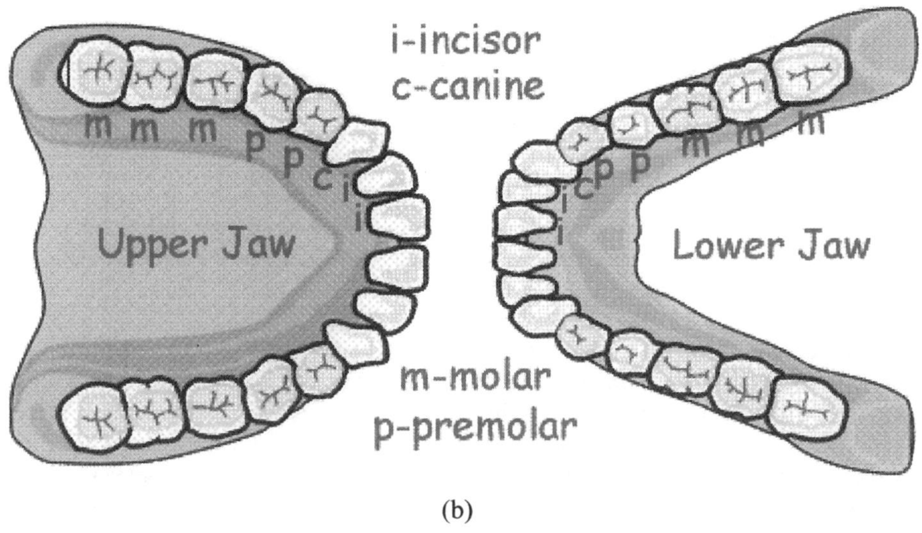

(b)

Figure 7.15 The structure and types of teeth (a) cross section through a tooth (b) the arrangement of the permanent or adult teeth

The diferent types of teeth are all designed to perform specialist tasks, as follows:– the 8 incisors (seizing and cutting food), the 4 canines (tearing tough roots &c.), the 8 bicuspids—or pemolars—(shearing and crushing), and the 12 molars (grinding and mashing).

Before considering the procedures for dental repair, we must understand how and why teeth decay. Teeth are at risk from acids in the mouth, which attack the calcium salts forming the main part of the tooth.. The most serious offenders are carbohydrates, especially sugars, which are converted by the micro-organisms in the plaque into lactic and other organic acids. Plaque ia the name given to the layer that forms on the surface of a tooth, primarily at its neck, and is composed of bacteria in an organic matrix. Plaque, incidentally, re-forms on the teeth as soon as the teeth have been brushed, but does not mature for 46 hours. The process of tooth decay is called "caries" and, if unchecked, will progressively destroy the crown and the pulp contained within it.

The use of materials in dentistry began with attempts to fill the cavities in the teeth, to prevent further decay and—before it is lost—to restore the profile of the crown, so as to allow it to function in the normal way. The earliest known fillings, used during the Middle Ages, were gums, waxes and resins. Towards the end of this period, many other materials—particularly lead and gold foil—were employed, gold being used as early as 1450. To begin with, it was considered sufficient simply to enter the cavity to remove the decayed material and insert the filling. After 1800, until about 1860, attention was given to modifying the cavity shape so that the filling would remain in place. From 1855, Robert Archer introduced the concept of "cohesive" gold foil, in which the metal was heated until its surface became pure, and was then cold welded into the cavity under mechanical pressure. Whilst this procedure, though tedious, gave satisfactory results; newer methods began to find favour. One of them, developed in 1828, was the silver amalgam. Silver, or one of its alloys, was mixed with mercury to form a paste, which was then pressed into the cavity.

In the light of the belief that the so-called "mercury poisoning" was harmful, not only when mercury was used in dental repairs, it was sometimes replaced by gallium and used with silver or tin alloys. Whilst a certain degree of stability was achieved by "undercutting" the cavity, improvements resulted from the use of a bonding agent to secure the amalgam to the dentine. An aqueous solution of a polymeric resin, such as HEMA (2-polyhydroxy methacrylate), was used to line the cavity, and the amalgam then inserted. By using both materials in the uncured state, intermingling occurred at the interfaces, and a mechanical bond resulted between the tooth and the filling.

Instead of using a liquid filler, especially where the cavity extended over a large area of the tooth, pre-cast fillings, or inlays, were used, and cemented into the cavity. The technique has essentially two variants; either metal posts are inserted into the expanded root canal, or screws and pins, are inserted into the dentine. Both act as the retention for an amalgam, or other filling materiald core, that can—like the stump of the tooth—be specially ground to the appropriate shape.

Whilst these procedures worked satisfactorily, cosmetically they looked like "metal fillings" and were generally not used with visible teeth. However, for some cultures the sight of gold-filled teeth were a sign of wealth and status!

The hunt was on for filling materials that not only were white enough for repairs to visible teeth, but which could also be tinted to match the colour of existing teeth. The technique eventually used was to "bulk-up" the known dental cements with fillers: usually powdered glass.

One of the earliest known dental materials—zinc phosphate cement, made by mixing a strong solution of phosphoric acid with zinc oxide powder—is still used for cementing (luting) metal crowns and crown posts in teeth. Zinc phosphate was followed by the silicate cements, which were actually used, not as cements, but as tooth-coloured restorative material. The silicates replaced coloured acrylic filling materials, and have themslves been replaced by glass ionomers, and resin-based glass composites.

In between zinc phosphate and the glsss ionomers, came the polycarboxylates, made from a mixture of zinc oxide and polyacrylic acid. Essentially these products, which are also based on phosphoric and polyacrylic acids, contain finely powdered glass fluxed with alumina and sodium fluoride. The function of the fluxes is to lower the melting point of the glass, and alter its chemical characteristics so that it is able to react with the matrix material.   Small quantities of trace metals are also used to create colour and opacity.

Today, the most widely used tooth-coloured filling materials are resin based glass composites   (filled resins) which comprise finely ground glass particles dispersed in an acrylic resin cured (cross-linked) by means of a suitable catalyst system. The overall properties of the material are, to some extent, controlled by the shape of the glass filler; just as the properties, and appearance, of concrete depend on the size and shape of the sand and aggregate, and the ways in which they pack in together.

Some recent work by Wolfgang Schaal in Germany, however has shown that zirconium oxide has many properties which are required as a dental material. Zirconium is superior in a number of ways to the more familiar ceramics. For example, it shows excellent biocompatibilty, and has high mechanical strength, combined with an exceptional crack-resistance. This latter property allows it to be used on its own, without bonding to a metal substrate, and also makes it possible to construct bridges (spanning several teeth).

From this short consideration of the tremendous range of dental materials, we can appreciate that the creation of these structures provides an excellent illustration of the principles of molecular architecture outlined in Chapter 2.

7.6.2. New Teeth for Old — Crowns

An alternative to the use of simple fillings or cast inlays, was the crown, or cap. This device is commonly available in two forms: plain metal and tooth-coloured. Tooth coloured crowns are available in the form of porcelain, usually bonded (fused) to a metal core, that is placed over the stump. Gold crowns are still used, or—in the case of the bonded crown—the metal is allowd to show through on the biting surface, because metal is less abrasive to the opposing teeth than porcelain. Although there are many different types of crown, a typical example is shown in cross-section in Fig 7.16

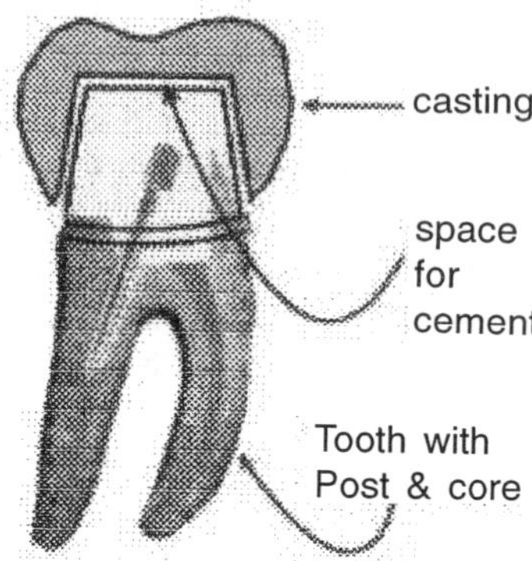

Figure 7.16 Cross-section through a typical dental crown

7.6.3. New Teeth for Old—Implants

Up to now we have concentrated on the repair of existing teeth, even though the use of crowns and caps sometimes entails the removal of large portons of the tooth. We must now consider how to replace a missing tooth (or teeth), or one which is so diseased that it has to be extracted

In the 18th century lost teeth were sometimes replaced with teeth extracted from human donors and forced directly into the vacant socket. As may be expected, the success rate was low due principally to rejection by the immune reaction of the recipient.

Over the next hundred years a variety of techniques were attempted. In 1809, a gold implant was placed into newly vacated sockets, and—after a suitable period for healing—a tooth crown was attached. In 1887, a physician named Harris used the same procedure with a platinum post instead of a gold one. The year before (1886) saw the implantation of a platinum disc into the jawbone, to which was attached a porcelain crown. More recently, at Harvard University in 1937, a series of implants made from cobalt-chromium-molybdenum alloy (vitallium) were tested, and did not suffer from rejection.

In 1952, a Swedish orthopaedic surgeon, Per Ingvar Branemark was doing research on the microscopic healing of bone defects in rabbits. His technique was to implant specially designed microscope heads—made out of titanium metal, with lenses mounted on the tips—into holes drilled in the thighbones of the anaesthetised animals. These were left in place so as to be able to photograph the healing process.

When the time came to remove them, he found that not only were they firmly fixed, but they were also completely biocompatible, and appeared to have integrated with the bone. He called this phenomenon "osseointegration", and now the use of titanium is commonplace in dental surgery.

Branemark's findings, together with those of other researchers, showed that it was possible to place a biocompatible implant into the human jaw in order to attach individual or groups of teeth, or as a scaffold for reconstruction work on the jaw. Whilst there are now many different implant techniques available, they can be categorised into three main groups:

* Endosseous Implants – Implanted directly into the jawbone
* Subperiosteal Implants – On top of the jawbone, but under the gum tissue
* Transosseous Implants – The fixing bolts penetrate the jawbone

A dental impant consists essentially of two main parts:

* The implant
* The abutment

The implant is a titanium screw inserted surgically into the jaw bone. When osseointegration has occurred, the second part can be connected. Since no two cases are alike, many different types and shapes of implants have been designed, each of which are inended to fulfil a particular purpose. The abutment, or post, fits into the implant and passes through the gum. It links the implant with the chosen prosthesis, which may be a single tooth, a multiple tooth bridge, or even a clip-on denture. Fig. 7.17 Illustrates a typical endosseous implant, and Fig. 7.18 shows some of the different implants discussed above.

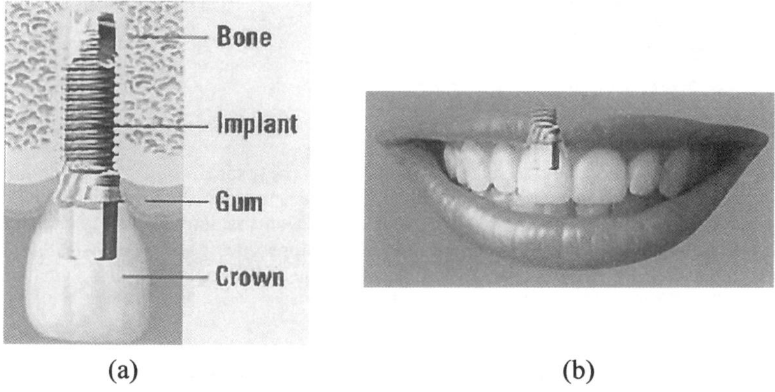

(a)   (b)

Figure 7.17 An endosseous implant (a) in cross-section (b) in place

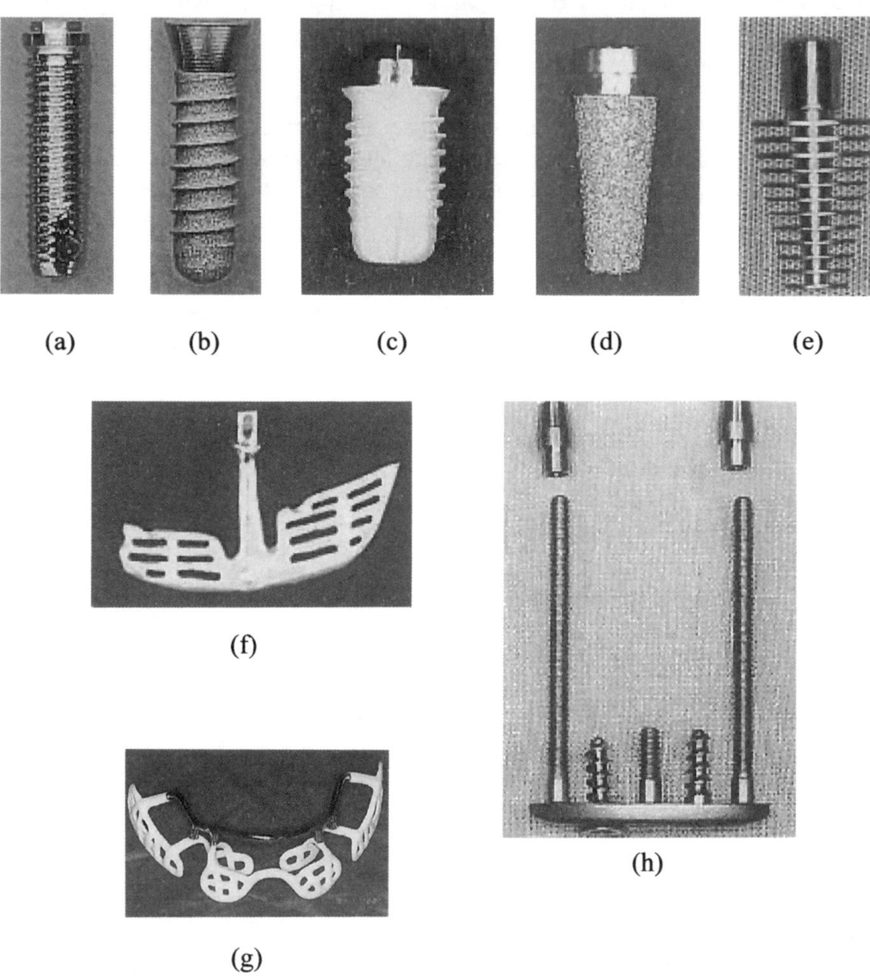

Figure 7.18 Types of oral implants (a) solid titanium implant (b) titanium implant with plasma sprayed surface to achieve greater bone integration (c) titanium screw implant with hydroxyapatite coating to promote osseointegration (d) tapered titanium implant coated with titanium beads (e) "Christmas Tree" designn (f) blade implant coated with hydroxyapatite for the upper jaw (g) a subperiosteal implant with hysdroxy apatite coating for the lower jaw (h) a titanium transosseous implant, which passe through the jaw

It is evident from the above that the design of implants, and the materials from which they are made, will provide the engineer and dental scientist with challenges for many years to come; especially in the provision of rapid and safely compatible prostheses.

7.6.4. New Teeth for Old — Dentures

There are occasions where the gaps saused by missing teeth can be filled without implants, but by a removable denture, or a plate on which are mounted the teeth necessary to fill the gap(s).

These are often made from a combination of plastics and metals, the latter used principally as reinforcing agents. The teeth themselves, which are embedded in a base structure, are generally made from acrylic polymers, sometimes cross-linked for greater strength. The body of the denture is usually made from PMMA, or a heat cured acrylic. Other materials, such as thermoplastic polyamides are also used. These are particularly useful in cases of allergic reaction to acrylics. Fig. 7.19 shows examples of full and partial dentures.

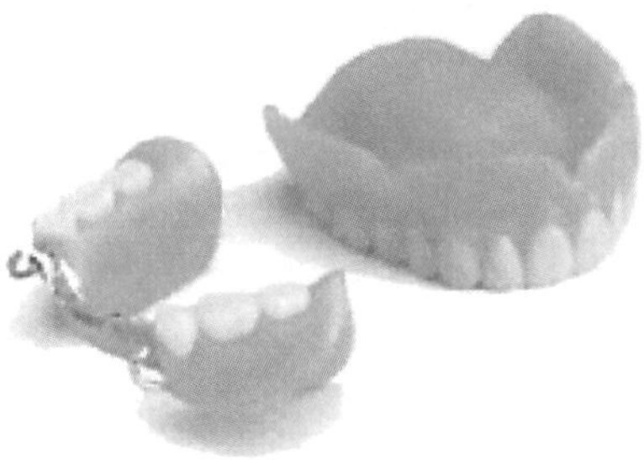

Figure 7.19 Examples of a full upper denture, and a partial lower denture

Where greater security is needed, dentures are sometimes fixed to implants in either jaw, and the dentures adhered by the inclusion of small magnets.

7.7. Reconstruction of the Jaw

Beyond the parts of the jaw containing the teeth, there are areas within the mouth where it is necessary to carry out reconstructive work: either from malformation, disease, accidental damage, or for purely cosmetic purposes. Again, as in the case of implants, a wide variety of materials and techniques is available, including the range of silicone elastomers, and the natural material—collagen.

Bone grafts are commonly used where areas of the jaw need to be replaced (see Section 7.5.2), and—as we shall see in the section on hip replacements—bone can be induced to behave in a plastic manner under sustained pressure. Called "distraction osteogenesis" the technique, pioneered some 50 years ago by the Russian orthopaedic surgeon Gavril Ilzarov, the techniques was used to extend leg bones, by inducing new cells to form under very slow extension.

The technique has been modified for facial reconstruction, and Dr Joseph G McCarthy, and his colleagues at New York University, have developed a three-dimensional tension inducing device for simultaneously correcting the height, length, and position of the jawbone (4).

7.8. Conclusion

It is evident from what we have discovered in this chapter, that—by using the correct material and appropriate design of the prosthesis—the problem of the interplay between materials and the body has been largely overcome. However, it must be realised that these successes have come largely as a result of compromise, and—in order to achieve greater perfection in many areas together—there are still many challenges to be solved by the engineer and the medical profession. Some of these I shall discuss in Chapter 9. In the meantime we must consider the role of implants under even more demanding conditions; the imposition of heavy loads or stresses.

References

(1) Sulzer Mitroflow Corp., Canada.; Mitroflow Synergy™PC.
(2) Ritchie R. O., *J. Heart Valve Disease.* **5** (1996), (Suppl.I): S9–S31.
(3) Mitka. M., *J. Amer. Med. Assoc.* Vol.283 No. 15 (2000), 223–234
(4) McCarthy J. G., *et al, Plastic and Reconstructive Surgery.* (2001), June, 564–566

Chapter 8

Load-bearing Implants

8.1. Introduction

We must now consider permanently implanted materials which are subject to considerable stresses, and which—from time to time—have to bear the full weight of the body, both at rest and in motion. These are replacement components for all or part of the different joints in the leg: the hip, knee, ankle and foot. Other such implants, which may have to suffer considerable stresses in use, but which normally do not have to bear the full body weight, are replacement joints in the arm: shoulder, elbow, wrist and hand

The major load-bearing joint replacements are generally used for older people, since those currently available tend to last for only about 15 to 20 years. Work is now under way to develop prostheses which can be implanted into younger, and consequently, more active people. These studies include determination of the most appropriate stress distribution in the femur and prosthesis, so as to give a close approximation to "normal" patterns.

One of the most interesting, and challenging, aspects of the design of artificial joints, is the behaviour of bone itself. Although, compared with other tissues in the human body, the bones seem to be quite hard and rigid, they are relatively easily deformed under pressure. There are numerous examples of enlarged or deformed organs, such as the liver, causing bone distortion, in which the bone—say of the spine—is broken down and reformed into a new shape (resorbed). It is also, of course, like most other living tissue, constantly being destroyed and renewed. As we have seen in the previous chapter, however, this phenomenon can be turned to advantage in the creation of new bone structures..

Although different in detail, the problems encountered in the design, implantation and survival of artificial joints are similar as far as the materials from which they are constructed, their behaviour in service, and the reaction of the body's immune system. It therefore seems sensible to deal with the individual joints separately, and then to consider matters which are common to them all.

8.2. Replacement Hip Joints.

The human hip joint comprises a "ball and socket" in which the rounded head of the femur is located in a cavity in the pelvic bone. Between the bones is a layer of smooth cartilage about 6 mm thick, which cushions the joint and allows the bones to move on each other with very little friction. When arthritis or an injury affect the

151

spacing between the ball and hip socket, making it painful and difficult to move the joint, it may be necessary to replace it with an artificial joint.

Artificial hip joints also comprise two main components working together: the ball and socket. Whilst attempts were made as long ago as the nineteenth century to replace joints which had become damaged by arthritis, the lack of suitable materials made the task almost insurmountable. Some ingenious solutions were tried, however, and I was recently shown a ball and spike, hand carved from ivory, which had been produced to solve the problem. The results were unsatisfactory, however, since the implant tended to split under stress, and break up.

In 1938, the British surgeon Philip Wiles (1896–1965), using stainless steel, produced a joint which showed promise, and—in the 1940s—the American surgeon Marcus Smith-Petersen (1896–1971) lined the bone socket with a polished steel cup, and reduced the diameter of the patient's femur so that it would fit into the cup. Two factors diminished the effectiveness of this solution: the tendency of the femur to jump out of the cup (dislocate), and the stiffness of the joint due to the friction between the bone and metal.

A more radical solution was adopted in the 1950s by two French surgeons, J and R Judet. They removed the corroded head of the femur, and replaced it with a plastic hemisphere mounted on a steel spike. This was inserted into the neck of the femur, and held in place with acrylic cement. The high level of friction between the socket and ball, however, caused the spike to work loose, making the whole joint unstable.

It was not until 1960 that the first successful prosthetic joint was introduced by the British Surgeon, Professor Sir John Charnley (1911-1982). Charnley spent most of his working life in his native Lancashire; graduated from Manchester University in 1935, and trained at the Royal Manchester Infirmary and Salford Royal Hospital. He began his research on hip replacement in 1954, financing his work with patent royalties from other inventions, including a "walking caliper" developed for wounded soldiers in World War II. After years of experimenting he found that the best combination of materials for a replacement hip was a thick plastic socket, and a small diameter highly polished metal ball to replace the head of the thigh bone. His original choice of plastic was PTFE, but this very soon wore out. He replaced it with a form of very high density polyethylene, which gave a joint with almost as little friction as the real thing. The socket and spike were secured in position by methyl methacrylate cement.

In 1961 Charnley opened a centre for hip surgery at Wrightington Hospital, Wigan, in Lancashire, where his methods are taught to surgeons of all nationalities. Today, more than 50,000 Charnley type hip replacement operations are performed annually.

8.2.1. Types of Artificial Hip Joints

Although there are many varieties of hip joint, there are essentially two main types: those that require bone cement to anchor them in the body, and those that do not; and —as we shall see later—there are important design differences between the two.

As is so often the case in surgical procedures, the precise choice of implant is made by the specialist, who needs to take account of a number of factors: these include the patient's age, lifestyle (how active the person is), whether the hip replacement is being done for the first time or is a replacement for a previous implant. The experience, training and personal preferences of the surgeon are also likely to play an important part, as is the observed condition of the bone components once they have been exposed. Additionally, robotics are finding an increasing role in perfecting this type of procedure (see Chapter 10).

Whatever design of implant is selected, it is highly probable that it will comprise a bearing made of a metal ball which moves inside a plastic cup. There are, of course, other materials—such as ceramics—which are used in some newer implants, and we shall consider them later. Fig. 8.1 shows some of the parts used in hip replacements.

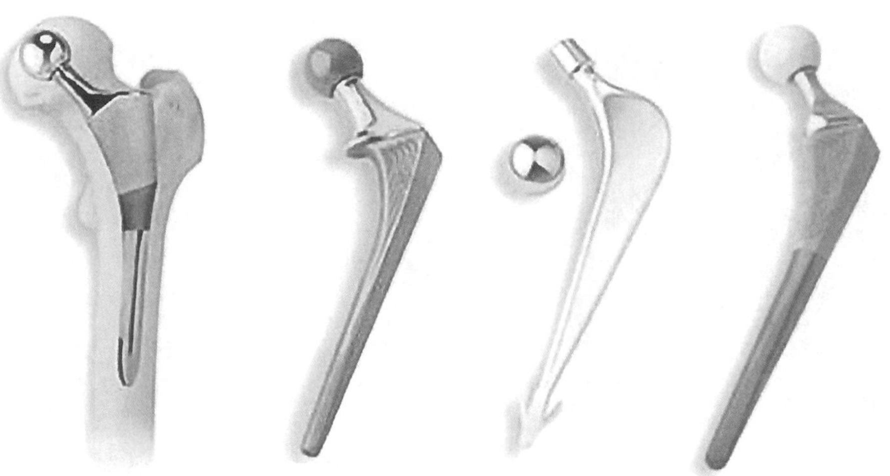

Figure 8.1 Different forms of hip stem used in hip replacement surgery (Courtesy Stryker Howmedica Osteonics, Allendale, New Jersey, USA)

Fig. 8.2 shows some cup and shell systems, and Fig. 8.3 gives an illustration of a completed hip replacement in both diagrammatic form and as an X-ray.

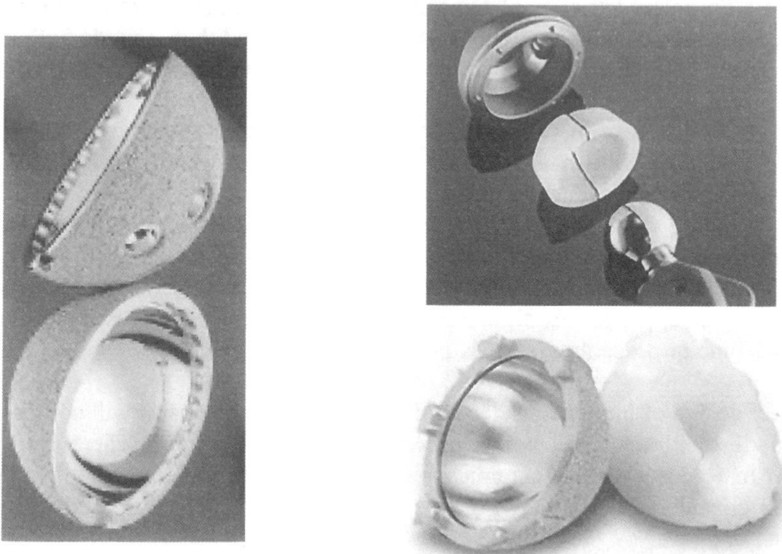

Figure 8.2 Illustration of different shell and cup systems for pelvic implantation (Courtesy B Braun Melsungen AG, Melsungen Germany)

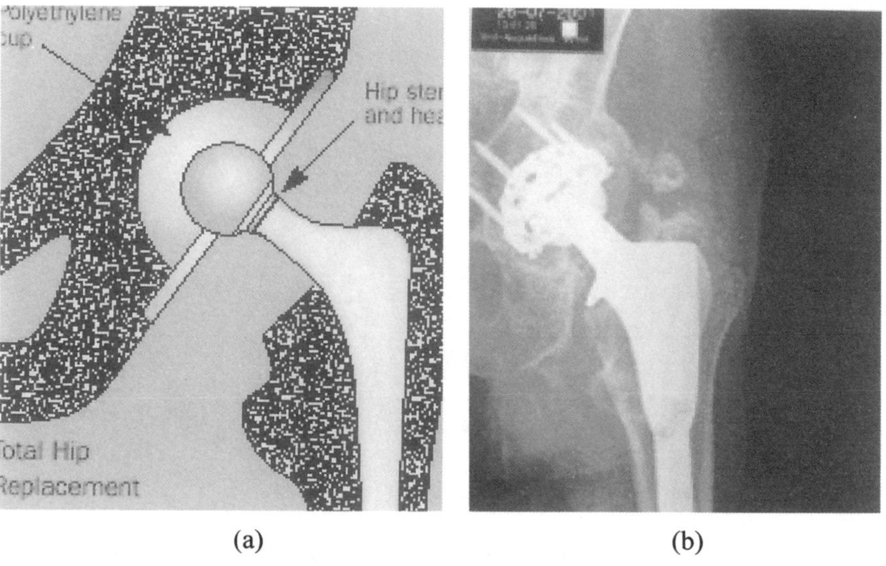

(a) (b)

Figure 8.3 Views of hip replacements (a) in diagrammatic form (b) an X-ray

8.2.2. *Factors Governing the Design of the Hip Joint*

Where synthetic implants are used in contact with bones, eg the hip joint, there is a greater chance of the prosthesis being successful if the blood supply to the rest of the bone remains intact, and the process of destruction and renewal can take place in the natural manner.

Of great importance, too, is the way in which the thrust is transmitted from the hip to the femur when weight is placed upon the assembly. As the imposed stresses are intermittent, and are applied from different directions, it is vital that the whole prosthesis is designed along sound engineering principles, and properly attached to the skeleton. The latter process, known as fixation, can be achieved with bone cement, or by new bone cells integrating with the metal of the hip prosthesis. (bone "ingrowth" or osseointegration)

In the case of the hip socket (acetabulum) the implant is generally made from metal (titanium or stainless steel), sometimes coated with a special ceramic material (hydroxyapatite), or roughened to promote bone growth, and comes in many forms: so that it may be cemented in place, screwed into place, or fixed with spikes or screws. Different types of lining: ultra-high molecular weight polyethylene or ceramic, are also available.

It is comparatively rare, unless the pelvic bone is weakened by disease, or damaged by accident (falling or crushing), for the cup to become loose or detached, and—since the hip remains essentially stationary against the movement of the femur— the stresses tend to be directed towards the centre of the cup.

In the case of the femoral stem, the range of stresses to be transferred includes:

* Compressive – taking the weight of the body when standing or walking
* Tension – bending or stretching
* Shear – twisting and turning

All of these cause loosening of the joint. Where there is simple mechanical contact between the bone and the implant, only compressive stresses can be transferred; in the case of the others, the pulling and twisting movements will loosen the joint. Also, unless the interfacial contact is complete, a fibrous membrane will form at the interface, causing further loosening of the joint. What is required is the development of continuity between the bone and the prosthesis. The metal surface alone cannot achieve this, since new bone will only form at a distance, before growing towards the implant. The use of acrylic cement certainly helps to generate a good bonding interface. However, where cement is not appropriate, the prosthesis is coated with hydroxyapatite, and new bone growth (osteogenesis) on the ceramic surface, begins to appear between the 5th and 7th day after implantation. In the same way as fracture healing, this growth is matched by reparative osteogenesis on the bone surface itself, and the bilateral ossification forms a bridge between the two surfaces, which is able to transmit forces, while at the same time is sufficiently elastic to absorb slight movements.

With cemented joints, high nitrogen stainless steel is generally preferred to conventional stainless steel or titanium, since the greater fatigue strength, resistance to corrosion and larger Young's Modulus (rigidity - see Chapter 2) tend to decrease the stresses in the cement layer. Recent studies have shown that tantalum is also biocompatible, and—when produced in the open form shown in Fig. 8.4—can encourage osteogenesis.

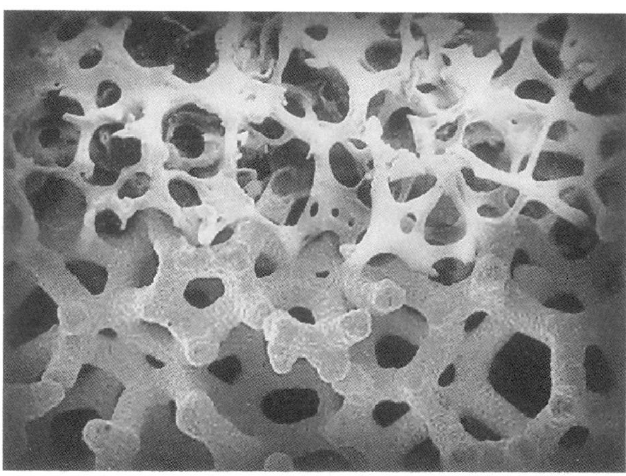

Figure 8.4 The open cage-like stucture of tantalum

Before we consider other work in hip replacements, it is appropriate that we should deal briefly with the subject of replacement knee and ankle joints, since many of the problems of design, materials and wear are common to most implanted joints

8.3. Knees, Ankles and Feet

8.3.1. Replacement Knee Joints

The knee is a "hinge type" joint, which is formed by two bones, the femur and the tibia, held together by flexible ligaments. The knee cap (patella) also forms part of the knee joint, and glides over the end of the femur as the knee bends. The moving parts of the knee are covered with a layer of articular cartilage. As in the case of the hip joint, either total or partial replacement becomes necessary when the normal function of the joint is impaired by disease or accidental damage. The procedure, known as Total Knee Arthroplasty (TKA), involves replacing the damaged cartilage, and resurfacing the bones of the knee joint with a metal and plastic prosthesis. Fig. 8.5 shows the normal knee, a selection of the components of a knee prosthesis, together with an illustration of a full joint replacement.

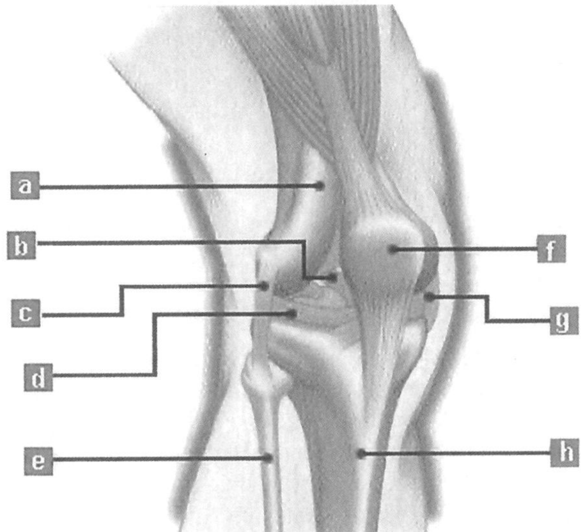

a Femur
b Anterior + Posterior
**   Cruciate Ligaments**
c Lateral Collateral
**   Ligament**
d Meniscus
e Fibula
f Patella
g Medial Collateral
**   Ligament**
h Tibia

(a)

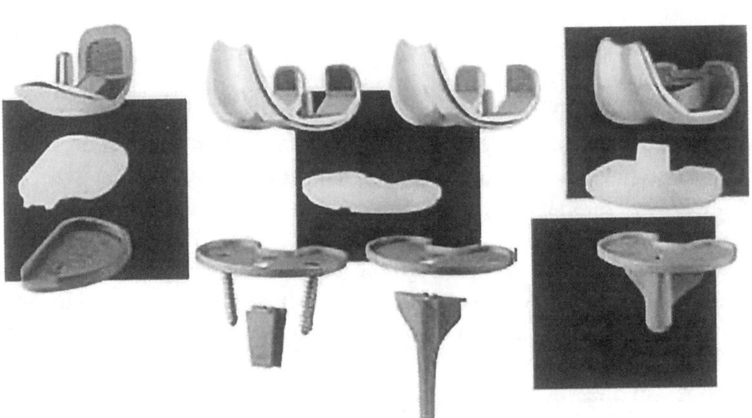

(b)

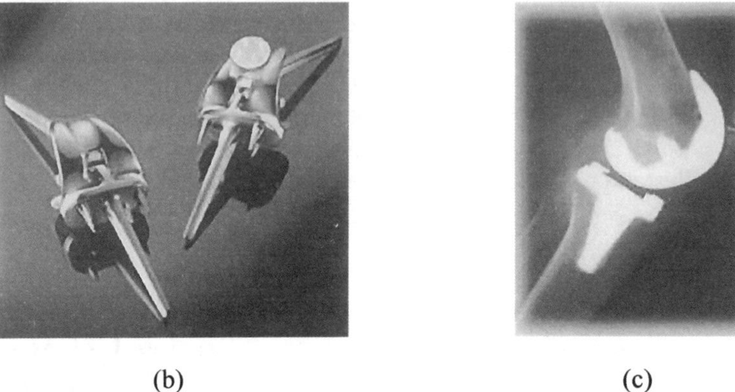

(b)   (c)

Figure 8.5 Knee replacements (a) the normal knee joint (Courtesy kneeindia.com) (b) the components of a knee prosthesis (Courtesy B Braun Melsungen AG, Melsungen, Germany) (c) X-ray of a total knee replacement

The pictures above illustrate typical modern knee replacement prostheses, and it is evident that the procedures involved are designed to remove as little of the damaged bone and tissue as possible, so as to enable the natural muscles and ligaments to play their normal roles. In the past however, there has been a tendency to seek an "engineering" solution rather than a biological one, so we find that many people have been fitted with devices that resemble the "universal joints" used in the motor and transmission industry! Certainly they work, but not as well—or in the same way—as the natural joint.

8.3.2. Replacement Ankle Joints

The ankle joint, unlike the knee and hip, has three bones at the junction—the tibia, the fibula and the talus (see Fig 8.6). It is also capable of more rotation and sideways motion than is the knee, and also—due to its smaller size—carries a proportionately greater share of the body weight compared with the knees and hips.

Consequently, until the late 1990s, the only method of treatment for severely damaged ankles (by arthritis or accident) was to fuse the joint, so that articulation was no longer possible. While this worked, and—to a large extent—removed the pain, the patient walked with a limp; and the unnatural gait transferred the stresses to the other bones of the foot. This unnatural gait, although allowing mobility and freedom from localised pain in the ankle joint itself, was the cause—in future years—of more extensive arthritic damage, and the whole situation became worse than before.

Although some 20 years ago there were about 8 different designs of total ankle replacement prostheses in use, the failure rate was high (over 50%), due to design faults and the failure of the cement used to secure them in place.

More recently, several new designs have appeared, and were successfully implanted in many countries; so far—after 10 years of implantation—over 80% of patients have reported pain free ankles. Although, as mentioned already, many designs and techniques have been tried out, the success of these new designs has been due to three main factors:

* The use of titanium nitride or cobalt chromium steel
* The meniscus bearing between the tibial and talar components is made from ultra high molecular weight polyethylene
* No cement is used to secure the joint components

The implants are generally 3 piece, and the metal components are coated either with titanium nitride beads or hydroxyapatite, both of which encourage bone ingrowth. The designs are also made more anatomically correct, by keeping the 9–11 sq. cm. bearing area found in the natural joint.

One of the most widely used ankle implants is the Agility™ Total Ankle System, made by DePuy, Inc., of Warsaw, Indiana. Fig. 8.6 shows the natural ankle and this type of prosthesis.

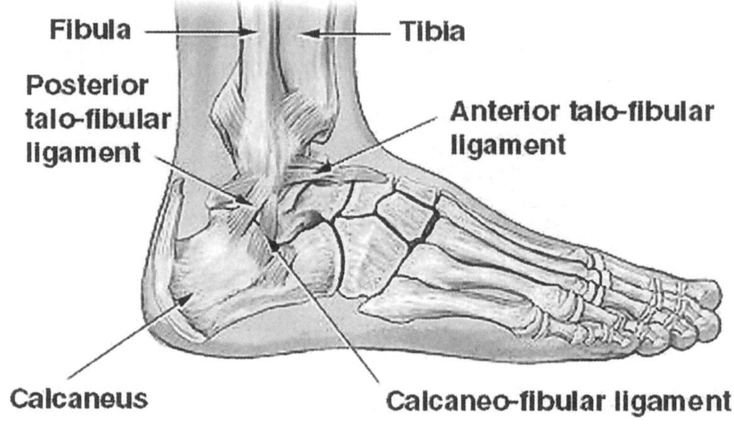

(a)

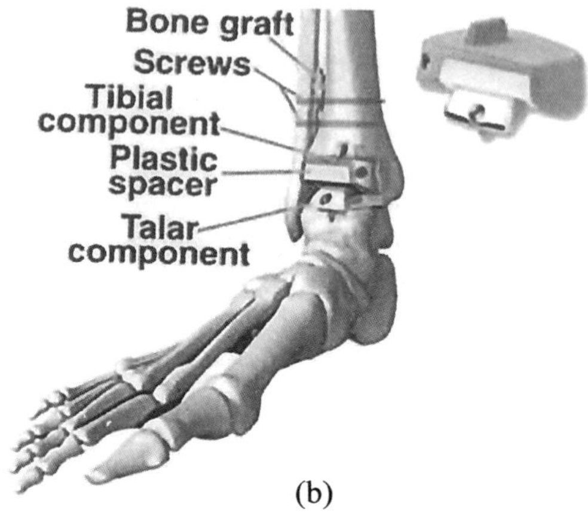

Figure 8.6 (a) The human ankle joint (b) the Agility™ Total Ankle Replacement System   (Courtesy DePuy Inc., Warsaw, Indiana, USA)

8.3.3. Surgery on the Bones of the Foot

The human foot is a flexible collection of soft, breakable bones. However, it is easily able to take the jarring weight of the whole body at rest, and in violent motion. It can do this, because the bones are encased, and held in place, by a web of sinewy muscles and ligaments possessing great tensile strength. (see Fig. 8.7) This structure spreads out the impact of the body weight through the tarsal bones, and the "arch" under the foot acts as a shock-absorber, while at the same time making it easier to walk.

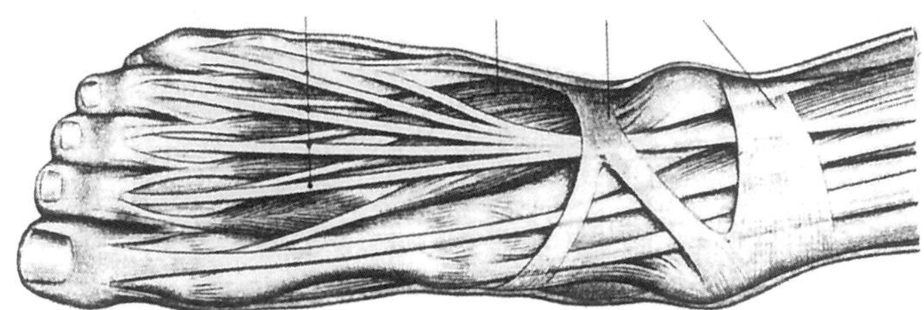

Figure 8.7 The muscles, ligaments and tendons surrounding the bones of the ankle

Replacements for the bones and joints in the foot have been in use for nearly 30 years.   The design of the implant and the materials used depend on which of the bones have to be replaced (size and function) and include polypropylene, ultra high density polyethylene, silicone elastomer, caramic structures cobalt/chromium/molybdenum alloys, as well as titanium/aluminium/vanadium alloys. Some examples of different toe joints are shown in Fig. 8.8.

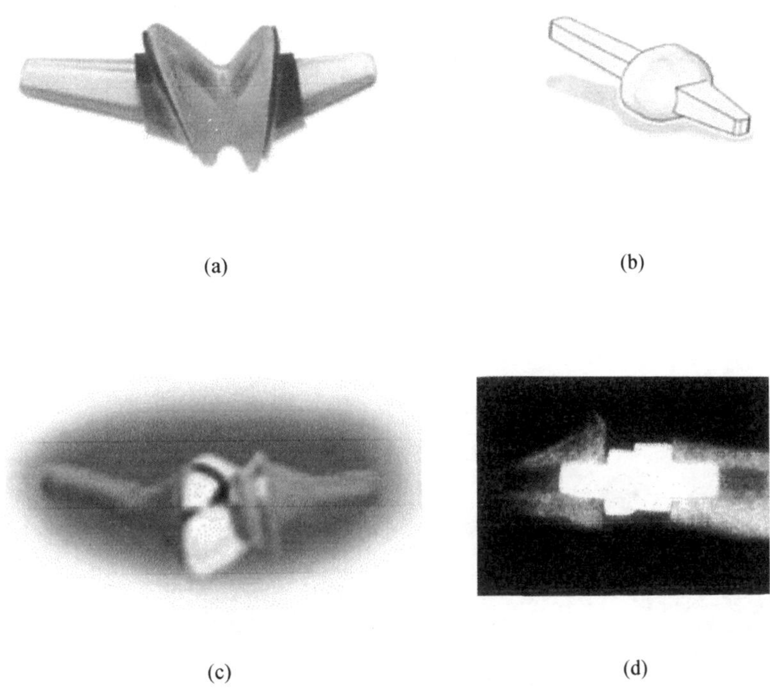

(a) (b)

(c) (d)

Figure 8.8 Some examples of different toe prostheses (a) silicone elastomer flexible great toe implant and (b) lesser toe implant (Courtesy Futura Biomedical) (c) metal/plastic hinged foot implant (Courtesy Osteo Tec UK) (d) ceramic "press-fit" implant Courtesy Orthosonics Ltd)

8.4. Shoulders, Elbows and Hands

8.4.1. Replacement Shoulder Joints

The shoulder, like the hip, is a complex ball and socket joint. It is also the joint which has the greatest mobility of any joint in the body, and relies for its stability on the muscle surrounding it (the rotator cuff), the capsule (a group of ligaments which connect the humerus to the scapula), and on the ligaments that attach the clavicle to the acromion (part of the upper spine) and also to the scapula. This is a complex, and consequently relatively easily damaged assembly, which is shown, together with joint replacement prostheses in Fig. 8.9.

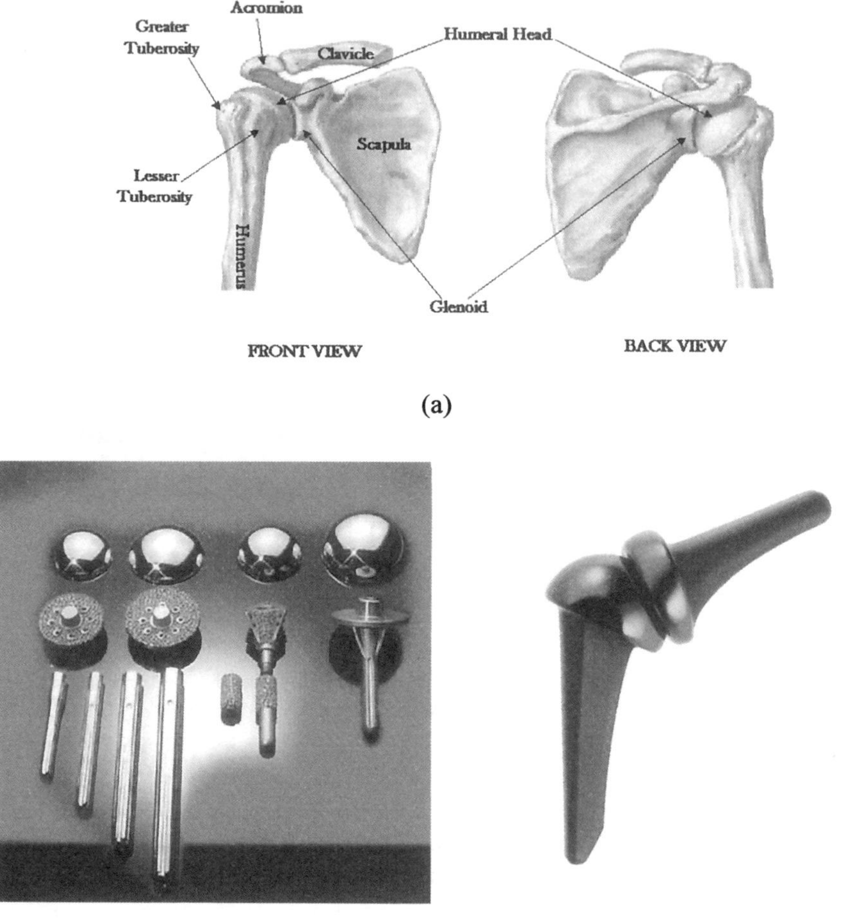

(a)

(b)

Figure 8.9 (a) the arrangement of the bones muscles and ligaments in the human shoulder (b) shoulder replacements.

As is the case with the other joints in the legs and arms, damage by injury or disease can also interfere with the smooth operation of the joint, and shoulder replacement (arthroplasty) may become necessary to restore function and remove pain. There are two types of shoulder replacement procedures

* Hemi-arthroplasty – where the upper arm bone (humerus) components only are replaced.
* Total shoulder arthroplasty (TSA) – if both humeral and glenoid (socket) are Damaged

Total shoulder replacement was introduced in the early 1970s by A C Neer, and others, including Harlan C Amstutz and Ian Clarke. The humeral component is intended to replace the humeral head, and is anchored by a stem inserted into the intramedullary canal (the hollow interior) of the humerus. Generally formed from alloys such as cobalt-chromium or titanium, it may be fabricated either as a single piece, or modular, with separate head, neck and stem components of different sizes and shapes.

The humeral stem may be fixed with bone cement, or simply press-fitted into the intramedullary canal, and a ceramic coating such as hydroxyapatite is often applied to encourage bone ingrowth. The concave glenoid component is generally made from ultra high density polyethylene, and fixed with bone cement. Because of the small surface area, it is vital to ensure that the bone/cement/prosthesis interface is as near perfect as possible.

8.4.2. Replacement Elbow Joints

As with the other joints in the body, the elbow is subject to damage by arthritis, both osteo– and rheumatoid–, believed to be caused by a disorder of the body's immune system (see Chapter 3). Accidental damage by injury is also fairly common, and for many years attempts have been made to develop a procedure for replacement of the joint. In the case of the elbow, however, replacement surgery is technically more difficult than hip and knee replacements, since the joint is smaller and more complex.

The earlier prostheses had a limited success rate, since surgeons had to choose between two implant types, each of which had disadvantages. The world's first successful total elbow replacement was performed by Dr Arnold-Peter Weiss, in 2001 at Rhode Island Hospital, USA. In this procedure, two metal implants were inserted, one into the end of each major bone connecting the elbow. A third component, joining the two other implants, was "customised" to meet the movement needs of the patient.

In an attempt to achieve the maximum reliability and mobility, many different designs have been produced: some with two prongs, some with three, and with many varieties of "hinge". Most were constructed from chromium or titanium alloys, with ultra high molecular weight polyethylene bearing inserts.. Two examples are shown in Fig. 8.10.

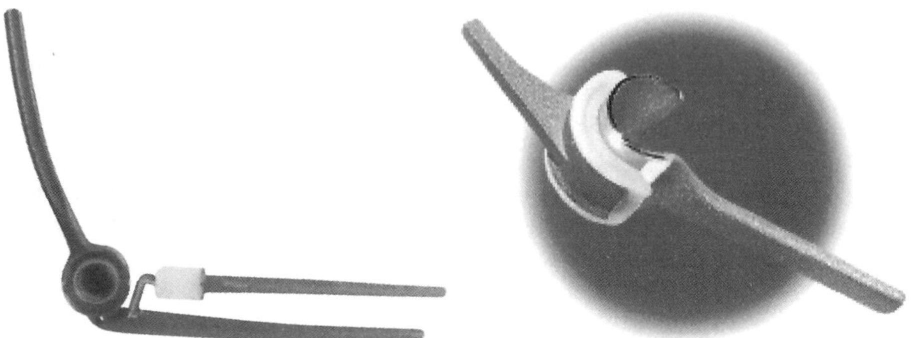

Figure 8.10 Examples of artificial shoulder joints

8.4.3. *Surgery on the Wrists and Hands*

As can be seen from the illustration in Fig 8.11, the wrist and hand is—to some extent like the ankle and foot—a highly complex structure, with a great many bones and individual joints, surrounded by a network of muscles, ligaments and tendons. This type of structure is necessary to perform the wide range of movements and functions required of the human hand.

One of the problems, however, in addition to the complexity of the joints, is their small size compared with the degree of strength needed for many of its tasks. Total wrist replacement has been carried out successfully using the type of prosthesis shown in Fig. 8.12.

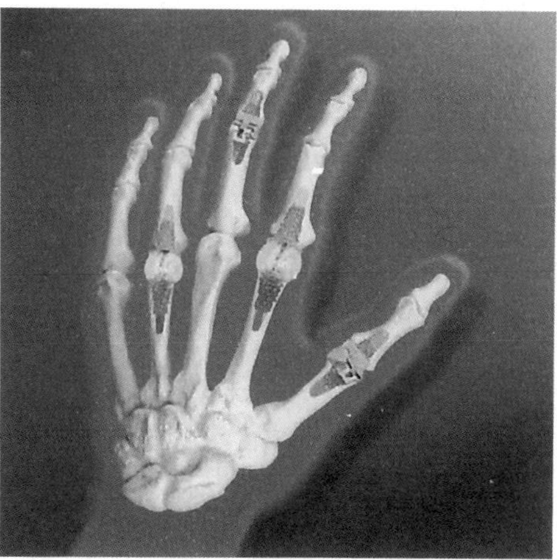

Figure 8.11 The bone structure of the human hand

The degree of movement and strength are good, but the patient has to agree not to do anything which causes sudden shocks, such as hammering, using pneumatic tools, skateboarding or rollerblading (because of the risk of falling).

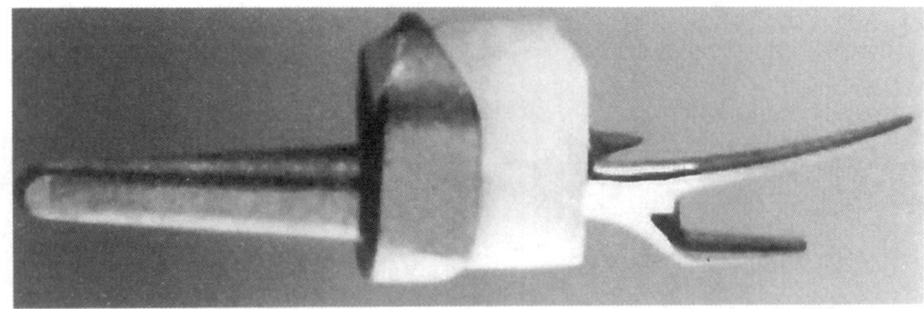

Figure 8.12 The Anatomical Total Wrist (ATW) system. (Courtesy University of Maryland Medicine, Maryland, USA)

It will have been noted in the illustraton of the bones of the hand (Fig. 8.11) implanted knuckle joints are in place. Finger implants have been used for over 30 years; the prosthesis being developed in 1969, after several years of research by Dr Alfred B Swanson, of Grand Rapids, Michigan, USA. The Swanson implant is made from silicone elastomer, and incorporates a built-in hinge. It is inserted into the bones on either side of the joint. Since the structure of the implant does not precisely replicate the biomechanics of the joint it replaces, it is normally possible only to achieve a range of motion roughly half of the 90 degrees in a normal hand. Fig. 8.13 shows examples of the Swanson finger joint, and some carbon prostheses; which have been successfully implanted. Work is currently in train at Durham University, England, on improvements to the design of the two component joint, which should allow enhanced mobility (1).

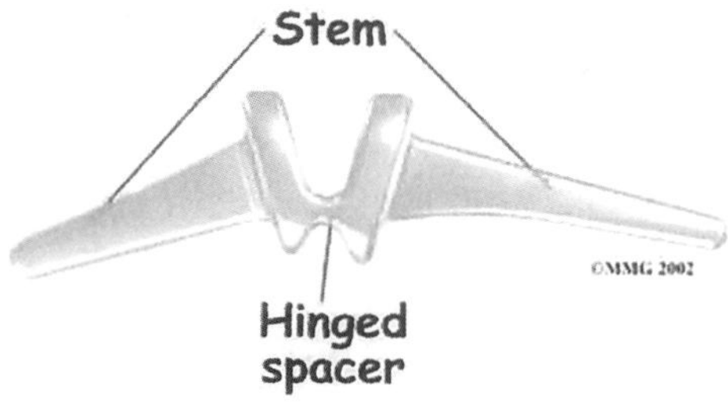

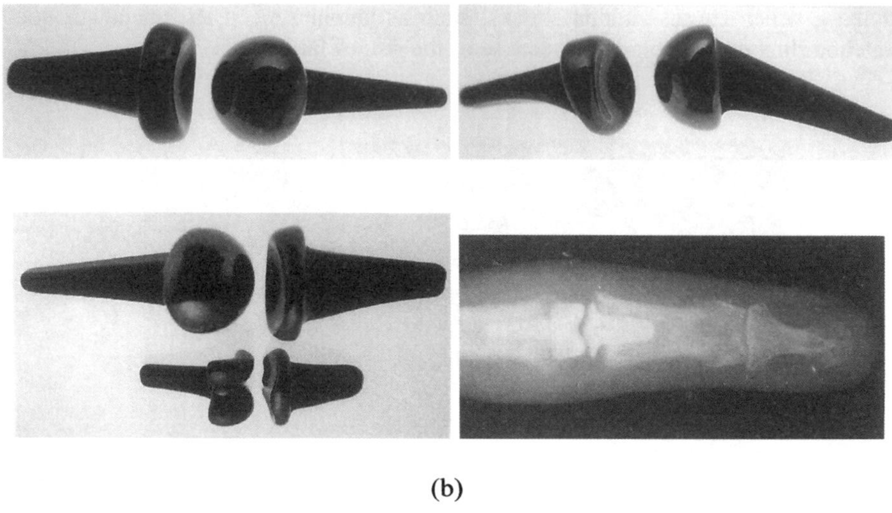

(b)

Figure 8.13 Examples of knuckle replacements (a) The Swanson Joint (b) some two component carbon joints, separately and in situ

If required during reconstruction, polymeric tendons may be temporarily implanted. These "rods" create a pseudosynovial sheath, which later lubricates and nourishes an autogenous graft.

8.4.4. *The Next Generation — Problems to be overcome*

Whilst the current generation of joint prostheses, in the main, give satisfactory results, there are still many topics which require attention, and which are being studied in universities, and by industrial companies throughout the world. However, diverse as they may be, it is possible to group them into three main categories:

*   Design
*   Materials
*   Performance

Design

In all of the areas discussed above, the quest in centres throughout the world has been to design prostheses that approximate more closely to the natural joint; this includes having two, instead of one articulation components (2). This not only has a more normal movement, but also decreases the stress on the polyethylene, which—in turn—reduces the amount of wear. In view of the decreasing age of patients needing replacement knees, studies are also in hand to design implants for the revision of failed implants (3). So as to keep track of the progress of knee and hip replacement implantations, national databases are being completed and co-ordinated worldwide (4).

Materials

In order to increase the durability of implant components, different surface treatments for metal parts have been evaluated, including titanium nitride (TiN, an extremely hard ceramic system with good adhesive properties. Cross-linked polyethylene has also been found to work well, and developments are in hand to improve the performance of a range of bone cements (5).

Performance

One of the main problems with artificial joints is the debris produced by the wear of metal/plastic, and sometimes metal/metal interfaces. The small particles produced have two adverse effects:

* They can interfere with normal working of the joint, and cause loosening
* As "foreign" bodies they are attacked by the body's immune system, and the chemicals so produced are also capable of attacking and destroying the natural bone

Many centres are investigating this phenomenon, including the Orthopaedic Research Unit in Cambridge University, England (6).

8.5. Conclusion

It is evident even from this brief treatment of joint repair and replacement surgery, that—particularly in the case of the smaller joints of the elbow, hands and feet—the surgical procedures involved are both complex and intricate. Also because of the structure of the joints, and the interplay of the muscles, tendons and ligaments, the problems of achieving strength and the maximum articulation are considerable.

It is not possible in a book of this size and scope to give more than an indication of the problems which are encountered with joint replacement systems, and the ways in which they are being tackled, but the field offers great opportunities and promise for partnership between many disciplines.

Tremendous advances are being made, even as this book is being written; some of them have been touched upon in section 8.3.4. Others, particularly in the fields of microsurgery, minimally invasive surgery, and the creation of new structures and materials, are introduced in Chapters 9 & 10.

References

(1) *Research Report, Dept of Engineering,* (University of Durham 2001)
(2) Bertini.G., *et al, Research Frontiers in Total Joint Replacement - B Knee Research 1.1* (Utah, 2001)
(3) Ibid. - *B Knee Research 3*
(4) Ibid. - *B Knee Research 2*
(5) Huddleston H. D., *Arthritis of the Hip Joint (2001)*
(6) Rushton N., *et al, Orthopaedic Research Unit, Publications,* (Addenbrooke's Hospital, Cambridge, 2001)

Chapter 9

The Tools of the Surgeon

9.1. Introduction

So far in this book I have concentrated on two main themes:

* The development of modern surgical techniques and medical procedures
* The properties of materials, especially plastics, and their ability to provide a solution to a tremendous range of medical problems

We have seen how the development of new and more sophisticated materials and engineering systems have made it possible for the surgeon to become more adventurous in operating on different parts of the body. At the same time the use of microsurgical and minimally invasive procedures allow advanced surgery to be carried out with less trauma to the patient, requiring shorter periods in hospital (or even day-care treatment), with consequent cost savings, and more rapid recovery times.

The creation of implantable materials which are more resistant to mechanical wear, eg ultra high density polyethylenes, and ceramics for joint replacements, high strength, lightweight materials for limb prostheses, and—above all—materials which remain functional in the hostile environment of the human body, have extended the surgeon's capabilities.

In metals, scientists and engineers at the University of Dundee, Scotland, are working on alloys which can adopt different shapes, depending on their temperature (1). One device that appears to show promise, is a suture, which looks like an office staple, and which can be made to close when heated by the passage of an electric current. This device is particularly useful in "keyhole" surgery, where delicate manipulations are essential, and where the recovery of the patient is achieved with minimal trauma.

Before we go on to consider some of the even newer "state of the art" surgical techniques, and the materials and processes which have made their development possible, we should take a slight pause and look back at the development of surgical instruments themselves; the tools of the surgeon. This idea was suggested, when reviewing the scope of this book, by one of the series editors who pointed out that a topic which could be of interest was the development of surgical instruments, as distinct from their use in surgery.

This seemed appropriate since, it forms a natural bridge between the use of materials in existing medical applications and the concept of the next chapter, entitled "Meeting New Challenges". Also, the type of instrument which can be created is strongly dependent upon the properties of the available materials, and the methods by which they can be fabricated into useful articles. The design element is also important, since—if a new material has been produced which has superior properties—it would be foolish, for example, to design a bronze knife resembling one made of flint. Having said that, though, the prime factors governing instrument design are, or should be, the requirements of the job to be done, and the needs of the person doing it. As we shall see later, it is interesting to note how an evolved design spans both the centuries and the different cultures.

Since, in the earliest times, it was believed that all illnesses were caused at a distance by gods, demons or spells, those concerned with the practice of medicine had no direct connection with the patient, but dispensed their curative skills from remote caves, or sacred groves. After treatment the patient was required to make a votive offering to the god who had effected the cure. Many disases were also tied to the concept of the four elements: earth, air, fire and water. These were identified as phlegm, blood, yellow bile and black bile, which had to be combined in the body in correct proportions. This idea, not of much use in itself, dominated European medicine for over two thousand years. Fig.9.1 shows a replica of the afflicted limb, complete with enlarged vein, offered in gratitude to the god for curing the suppliant's varicose veins. The figure also shows a 14th century illustration of the four humours.

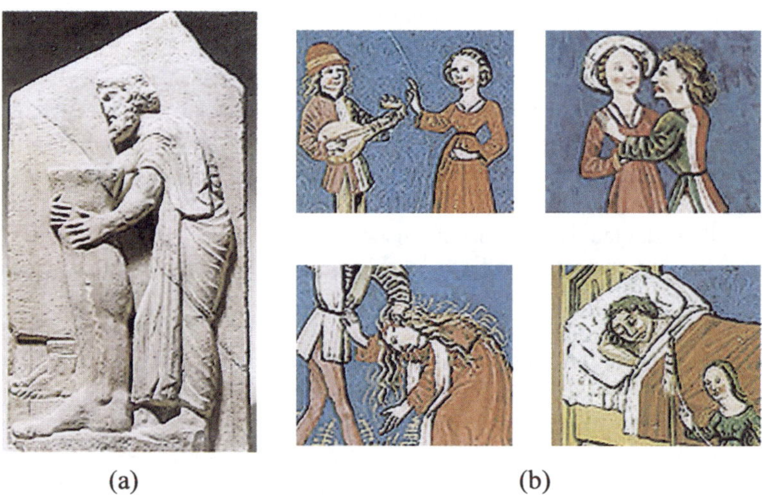

(a)   (b)

Figure 9.1 (a) a votive offering to Asclepius (b) the four humours

It was not until the development of writing, some 8,000 years ago, that the description, diagnosis, and cure of ills could be written down and documented. Some 5,000 years ago, the walls of caves and buildings in Egypt depict an impressive array of surgical instruments, easily recognisable as the forerunners of some of those in use today.

Many years were to elapse before the concept of a direct "hands on" aproach was adopted, and the remedies used were often both brutal and drastic! Fig 9.2 shows some of the procedures.

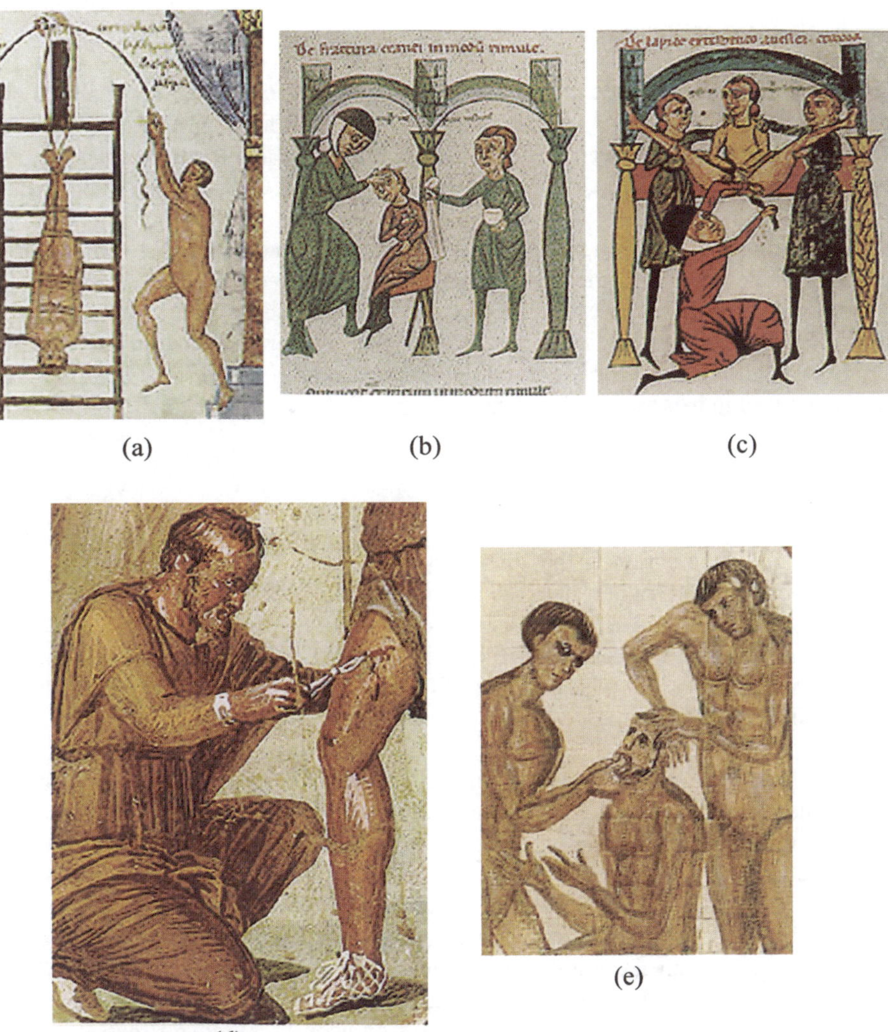

Figure 9.2   Some early treatments of wounds and illnessesses (a) treating dislocations by jolting on a ladder (b) surgical   examination of a fractured cranium (c) operation for bladder stones (d) Aeneas receiving attention from Iapys (e) bone setting of the jaw

After this brief introduction it would, I think, be logical to start with the simplest tools, like the flint scalpels recently discovered in Colchester, England—and used more than 2,000 years ago (2)—and to progress towards technologies so sophisticated that they involve the synthesis and handling of materials a thousand times thinner than a human hair!

9.2. Early Surgical Instruments

The variety of materials used in surgical instruments is tremendous; starting with the natural materials like stone, shells, wood and animal horn, progressing through bronze, copper, iron and steel, to the newer metal alloys, and thence to plastics, and the harder materials such as ceramics, tungsten carbide (WC), and even diamond.

Interestingly enough, there are many museums around the world with galleries and libraries devoted to surgical instruments; and the collection of early examples as an art form has become an established part of the antiques business, particularly in the United States. As we shall see later in the chapter, the instruments devised during the 19th century, for use in battle, are particularly elegant and compact, and are also housed in handsomely lined cases.

9.2.1. The Ancient World

We have already mentioned the discovery of flint tools which, seemingly, were intended for medical rather than domestic use: the Bible records circumcisions carried out with flint knives. There is also evidence that wood and horn implements were used. At about the same time, other ritual operations, amputations and entry to the skull, were carried out with stone and flint saws, as well as with obsidian—which could be flaked to almost molecular thinness.

Later on, however, the overwhelming majority of early surgical instruments were made of metal. In the Roman Empire, and in Greece, most instruments were made of bronze, or occasionally silver. Iron was rarely used because, as in most ancient cultures, it was considered taboo by both the Greeks and Romans, and so was never used for surgical instruments on religious grounds. One of the most fruitful sources of ancient Roman instruments was in the so-called "House of the Surgeons" at Pompeii. Although the number of surgeons' shops is sufficient to suggest that some physicians specialised in surgery, there was some distinction—even if not a rigid one—between general practitioners and surgeons. Medieval texts, too, use different terms for the two roles: "medicus" for a doctor, and "magister" for a surgeon. Fig. 9.3 shows a Stone Age trephination saw (for removing a circular piece of tissue or bone, generally from the skull), and two steel instruments used in England during the late middle ages.

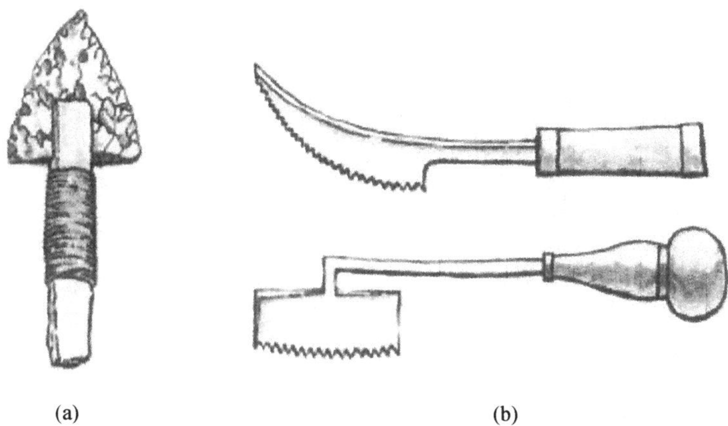

(a)　　　　　　　　　　　　　　　　(b)

Figure 9.3 Early surgical instruments, (a) a flint trephination saw (b) two English steel trephination saws with brass-bound wooden handles

Fig. 9.4 shows some examples of the variety of instruments excavated from the ruins of Pompeii (3) .

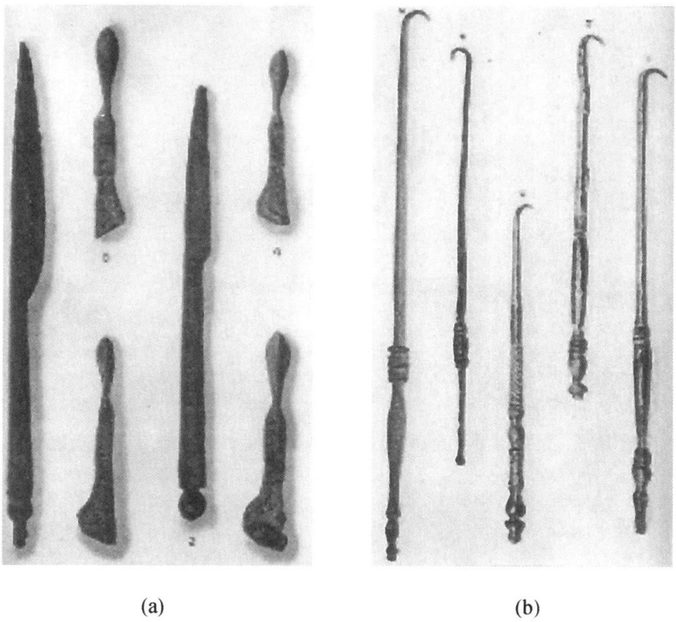

(a)　　　　　　　　　　　　　　　　(b)

          Life-enhancing Plastics

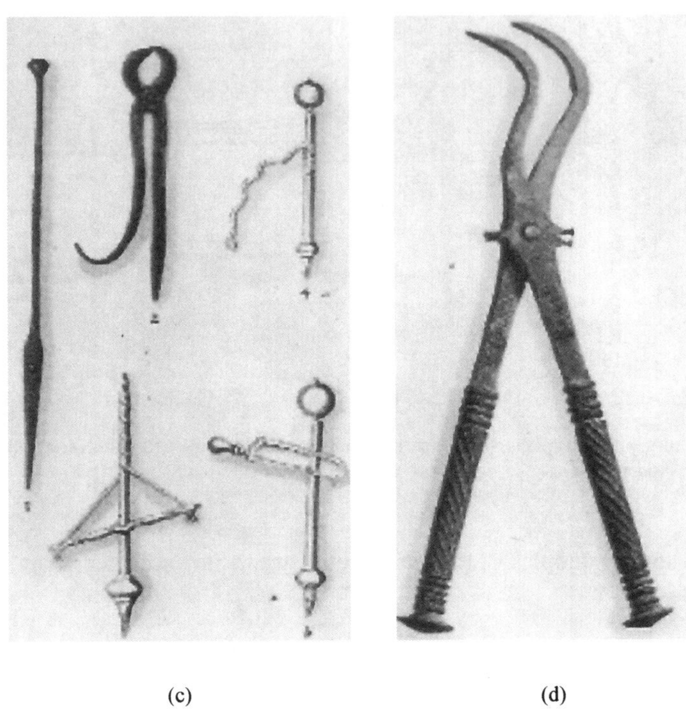

(c)   (d)

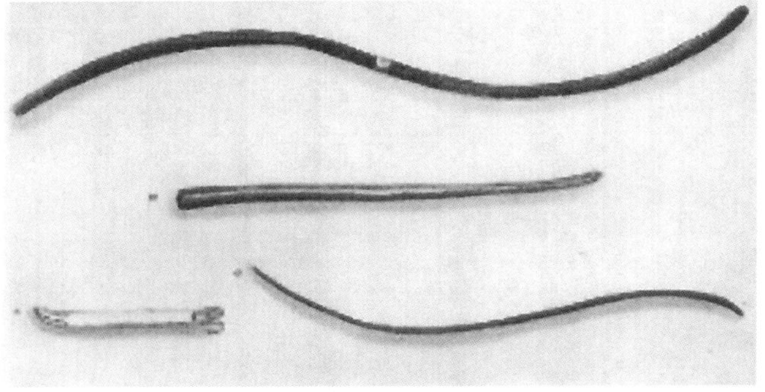

(e)

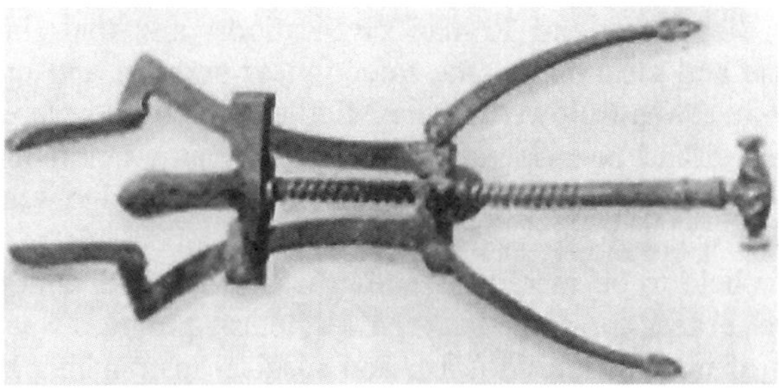

(f)

Figure 9.4 Instruments excavated from the ruins of Pompeii (a) scalpels (b) artery hooks (c) bone drills (d) bone forceps (e) urethral catheters (f) vaginal speculum

Stone carvings and early paintings show that surgery was also practised in other ancient civilisations: including Egypt, Japan and throughout Islam. In the case of Islam, much of the knowledge came from the study of Greek and Roman texts, and then found its way into Europe.

The Chinese believed that disease could be cured by the restoration of harmony and balance between the five basic elements of earth, water, fire, wood and metal. However, as human dissection was forbidden in ancient China, physicians knew nothing about surgery (and, because of the way they treated illness, little about anatomy).

In Indian medicine, by contrast, surgery was widely used, and almost all major operations were performed by the Ancient Hindus nearly a thousand years before they were practised by the Greeks. Indian surgeons used more than 120 different steel instruments to sew up wounds, drain fluid, remove kidney stones and to perform plastic surgery. As an official punishment for adultery was to cut off the offender's nose, Indian surgeons had plenty of opportunities for the reconstruction and refinement of noses!

This vigorous discipline is mirrored by the Mesopotamian king Hammurabi (c. 1792-1750 BC), who ordained that "If a doctor has treated a nobleman with a metal knife for a severe wound, and has caused the man to die, or has opened a nobleman's tumour with a metal knife, and destroyed the man's eye, his hands shall be cut off." A stern penalty for medical malpractice, which would make it difficult to continue to practise!

9.2.2. *The Next Thousand Years – (500–1500 AD)*

The decline of the Greek and Roman civilisations, and their high standards of
surgical expertise and cleanliness (the infection of surgical and other wounds was
relatively unknown), was followed in the Middle Ages by a severe deterioration in
surgical knowledge, and post-operative infection became common. This was due
largely to the fact that most of the medieval medical knowledge was based on Greek
and Roman texts, which were available only to members of the church. As the
human body was held to be sacred dissection was prohibited, and had to be carried
out by the "lower orders" or surgeons. Nevertheless, progress was made especially
in the treatment of wounds and injuries; and surgical instruments included scissors,
speculum, razor, scalpel, needle and lancet.

In the 10th century Abulcasis of Cordoba (also known as Al Zahrawi) wrote a
monumental treatise on medicine and surgery. He designed over 200 surgical
instruments, some shaped like miniature scimitars, and many of them highly
decorated. These were used to operate on, among other things, diseased tonsils,
ophthalmic cataracts, the thyroid, bladder, limbs, abscessed teeth and haemorrhoids.

A page from this work is reproduced in Fig. 9.5, together with a decorated
bronze trepanning instrument from a slightly later period (ca 1200– 1400).

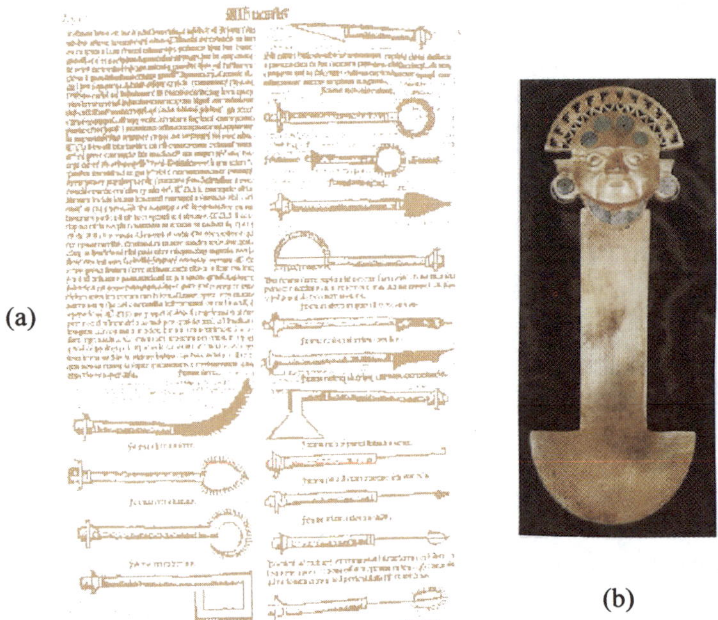

(a)

(b)

Figure 9.5 Early surgical instruments (a) from a manuscript by Al Zahrawi (b) Bronze trepanning knife

As we saw earlier, the actual practice of surgery in medieval times was carried out mainly by assistants, and it interesting to note that the design of many of the instruments then in use resemble those that would have been used by tradesmen, such as carpenters, butchers and cobblers. These can be seen in Fig. 9.6, which shows a drawing by Ambroise Paré (1510–1590). However, as the surgeon's centre of attention moved away from dissection of the dead to the treatment of the living, the design of surgical instruments changed from those of the tradesman to the medical specialist.

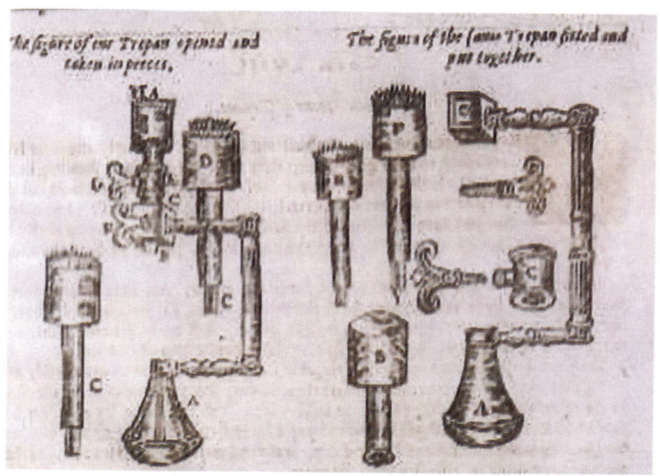

Figure 9.6 A page from "Dix Livres de la Chirugie" (1564) by Ambroise Paré

We must remind ourselves that despite the very considerable advances in knowledge and techniques, surgery remained a pretty awful experience, carried out in unsanitary conditions with no anaesthetic, and often with little skill.   Fig. 9.7 shows a 19th century trephination (trepanning) instrument, and Fig 9.8 shows the process itself—little changed over several thousand years, except for the positioning device.

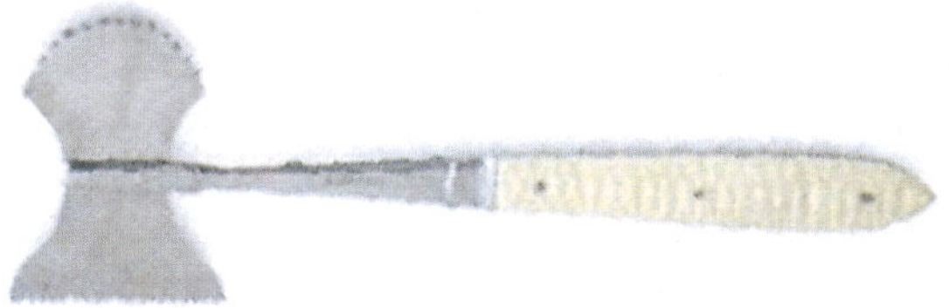

Figure 9.7 A 19th century trephine saw

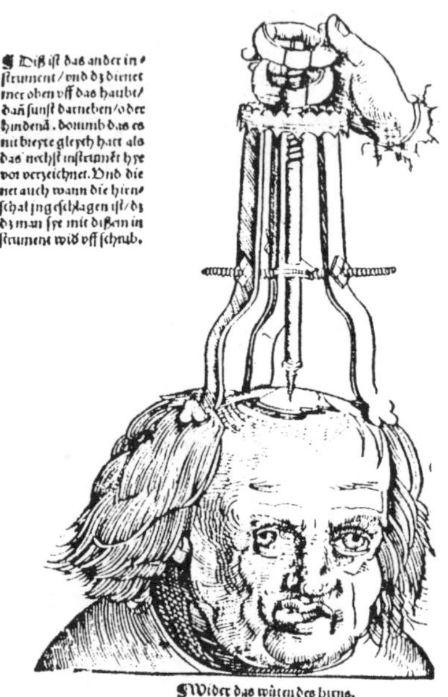

Figure 9.8 Trepanning, the medieval way, Hans von Gersdorf (1517)

9.2.3. *Four Hundred Years of Progress – (1600–1900 AD)*

The next four hundred years, following the Reformation, saw tremendous changes in surgery and surgical techniques, largely due to two important events. The first was the observation, in 1603, by the English physician William Harvey (1578–1657), that the blood circulates through the body as a result of the beating of the heart (4). The second was the birth of the industrial revolution in England, which began in about 1760, and which gave the means of creating new and improved materials, as well as the fabrication of tools and instruments in large, reproducible, quantities.

The 17th century also saw the invention of the microscope, which allowed surgeons to examine and treat anatomical structures which had not been exposed to study before. This, of course, demanded the production of finer instruments to deal with them. However, although these developments saw the refinement of existing designs, there was virtually no fundamental innovation; indeed, the surgeon of today would be quite at home with instruments produced some two hundred years before, and would probably admire those produced in the mid-1800s with their polished brass fittings and ivory handles, all housed in plush and satin lined leather and wooden cases. Some examples of these eagerly sought-after collectors' pieces, both "grooming" and surgical, are shown in Figs. 9.9 & 9.10.

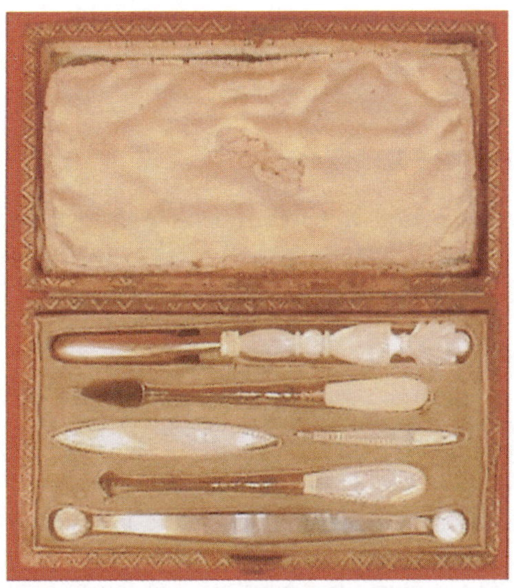

Figure 9.9 A gentleman's dental hygiene set (c.1780–1800). The set consists of a toothbrush, two scalers, a folding toothpick, a spool for holding floss, and a tongue scraper with silver blade. The spool is made of decoratively carved mother-of-pearl, and the instruments have carved mother-of-pearl handles. The set is housed in a gold-tooled red leather hard case, which contains a mirror, protected with silk-covered padding (Courtesy Alex Peck Medical Antiques, USA)

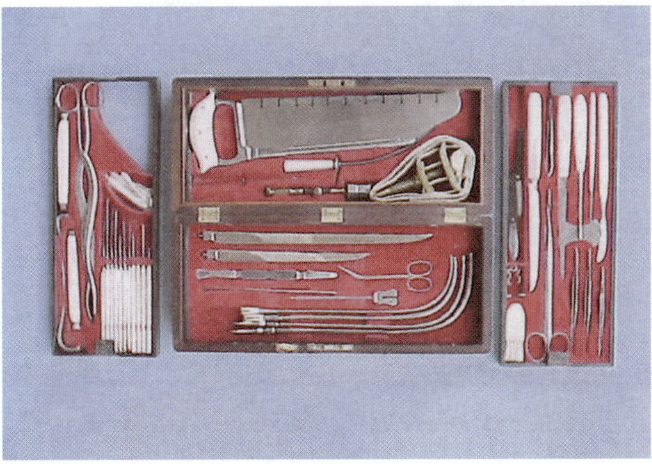

Figure 9.10 Part of an ivory handled, four tier, amputation set by George Tiemann of New York, USA, (c. 1850) (Courtesy Alex Peck Medical Antiques,USA)

The writing was on the wall, however, because the newly discovered benefits of steam sterilisation would have caused the delicate inlays and ivory handles to split and perish, and the animal glue which held them together to dissolve. Since stainless steel and other alloys were not universally used, the problem of corrosion was also of some importance.

9.2.4. *The Twentieth Century*

The 20th century was a period when considerable change took place in the design and manufacture of surgical instruments, as well as the materials from which they were made.

Two of the most significant advances were:

* The development of highly sophisticated specialist sets
* The introduction of plastics and ceramics

Whilst we have seen that many surgeons in the 19th century used "surgical kits", these were usually compiled to undertake a series of specific procedures, often on the battlefield. In the 20th century, however, we see the introduction—design, manufacture and marketing by specialist firms—of surgical sets intended for specific purposes, and containing many individual pieces. Fig. 9.11 shows a brief panoramic view of some modern surgical instruments.and devices.

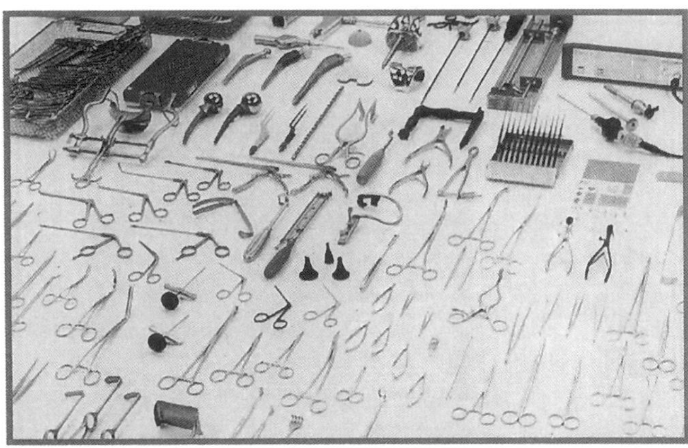

Figure 9.11 An array of surgical instruments and devices

Thus we find that one of the major suppliers of surgical instruments (Sklar, of West Chester, Pennsylvania), offers no less than 29 different surgical sets, with some containing more than 60 items. It is interesting to note that there are 28 different types of scissors in the product list. When one remembers that a busy hospital must be able to perform many different operations in several theatres, it is clear that the instrument store must be able to acommodate several hundred, or even thousand, sets; this in itself a costly investment in terms of purchase, space, maintenance and repair.

It is evident that such a complexity of applications will need, not only highly specialised designs (some of them, admittedly like the human body, not much changed over several thousand years), but also a careful tailoring of material properties. Apart from specialised, and disposable instruments, the great majority of reusable and sterilisable surgical instruments are made from stainless steel. The methods used to create the required properties are a good example of the principles we considered in Chapter 2.

Stainless steel, developed in England in about 1903, owes its "stainless" quality to the presence of a relatively high proportion of chromium (12–18%), and the excellent corrosion resistance is due to an invisible, passive oxide film that forms on the metal's surface in air. Many varieties of stainless steels also contain small quantities of carbon, nickel, sulphur, tungsten, manganese and molybdenum. Carbon is a prime consideration in instruments which require extremely sharp edges, or accurate jaw geometry.

Instruments are made from metal bars in the following stages: forging, fitting and polishing. With better quality instruments, these stages are carried out individually—often by hand. At the fitting stage, serrations and profiles are cut with special milling cutters, the components fitted together, and ground to size; after which they are correctly set, a vital operation in, for example, the case of pressure forceps.

After the fitting stage the instruments are still "soft", and have to be hardened and tempered. by heat treatment. Hardening (at about $760^0 - 870^0C$), followed by quenching in water or oil, sets up large internal strains in the metal, which have to be relieved by tempering, or annealing. This process results in a decrease in hardness and strength, and an increase in ductility and toughness. The primary purpose of the heat-treating process is to control the amount, size, shape and distribution of the carbon particles in the steel, which, in turn determines the physical properties of the material (see Chapter 2).

The use of inserts made from the extremely hard metal tungsten carbide (WC) not only provides exceptional hardness in needle holders and scissors, but also enable the parts to be replaced when worn. In addition to giving durable cutting edges, the hardening process—when suitably controlled—can give a measure of spring to retractors so that the surgeon can "feel" the conditions placed on the instrument. The spring that returns a handle back to its position is also made from the same material as the instrument itself, but specially hardened to retain its shape.

The appearance of plastics, both thermosetting and thermoplastic, which could be moulded into handles—either directly onto the blades, or separately for subsequent attachment—opened another chapter in the design and manufacture of surgical instruments. Again, their downfall was the use of heat and steam sterilisation. The gradual introduction of disposable scalpels; with metal blades fitted into moulded plastics handles, and supplied in radiation sterilised packs, alongside a whole range of tweezers, clamps and other instruments, which were discarded after being used only once, made further inroads into the supremacy of all-metal tools. Some single-use disposable surgical instruments are shown in Fig. 9.12.

(a)

(b)

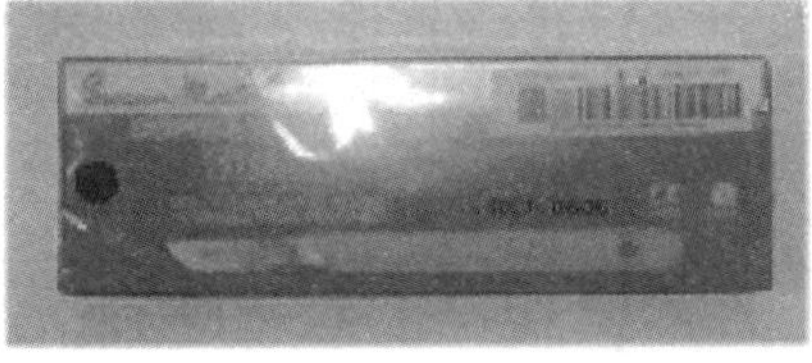

(c)

Figure 9.12 Disposable surgical instruments (a) stitch cutters by Ribbel International Ltd, UK (b) disposable scalpels by George Tiemann, USA (c) Swann Morton disposable scalpel blades in sterile pack; supplied by Westons Internet Home Health .

The range of modern surgical instruments is enormous, with special designs for every conceivable function; including clamping, opening, closing, cutting, and the whole range of metals, plastics and ceramics has a role to play.

The evolution of microsurgical techniques, and minimally invasive surgery, fuelled the development of instruments which took up very little space, could be made with great precision, and—where necessary—could navigate along intricate passages within the body. The coming of robotics also added a further dimension to the design of instruments, many of which owed their success to experience gained in the space industry.

9.3. Conclusion

This brief discussion of the development of surgical instruments from the earliest times to the present day has led us to three main conclusions:

* The fact that as the human body has remained virtually unchanged over the period, the design and function of many of the earliest instruments are easily recognisable today
* The design and manufacture of surgical instruments has progressed from those of the tradesman to the surgically competent specialist
* The development of surgical instruments was constrained to follow the availability of new materials from which the required properties could be obtained.

Now, in the next chapter, we must turn to the use of surgical instruments and techniques in an even more sophisticated environment, where extremely exacting requirements have to be met.

References

(1) Cuschieri Sir A, et al, Surgical Skills Unit, University of Dundee, Newsletter 2003
(2) Discover, (Gale Group) 1998, March, page 1
(3) Milne J S, *Surgical Instruments in Greek and Roman Times.*Clarendon Press, 1907
(4) Harvey W., *Anatomical Study of the Motion of the Heart and of the Blood in Animals,* 1628

Chapter 10
Meeting New Challenges

10.1. Introduction

In the last chapter, having considered the development of surgical instruments in the light of the materials available at the time, and—having regard to the requirements of the surgical procedures to be undertaken—we became aware of the extent to which the frontiers of surgical capability were being pushed back by new developments in a variety of different disciplines. These included physics, engineering and chemistry, all of which led to the development of machines and instruments which were capable of carrying out tasks with greater precision, and on a smaller scale than had hitherto been envisaged.

These are sensational achievements, and the rate of advance over the last few years has been quite breathtaking; in fact some of the surgical techniques which I have described earlier in the book have, during the writing, become modified, or extended, by the development of new techniques and procedures. Some of these we shall consider later in this chapter. It would, I think, also be appropriate to "peer round the corner" in order to see if we can forecast what other advances there are likely to be in materials, and their consequences for medical applications. We shall also look at some of the exciting new developments in the field of natural materials and polymers.

Among other topics I want to consider, are surgical interventions on a very small scale, the increasing use of robotics, and the exciting new world of nanotechnology (one thousand millionth of a metre) in which we can literally tailor-make new biocompatible materials on the molecular scale. This is where polymers really come into their own.

10.2. Minimally Invasive Surgery

We have already, under the review of different surgical techniques, touched upon the use of small-scale interventions, and their benefits, both to the patient's speed of recovery, and to hospital economics. It is now appropriate to deal briefly with the subject in rather more detail.

First, it would be helpful to make the distinction between microsurgery, "keyhole" surgery and minimally invasive (or minimal access) surgery. As we saw in chapter 1 microsurgery is concerned with the performance of extremely intricate operations, using highly refined magnification systems, and very small instruments. The technique enables the surgeon to gain access to previously inaccessible parts of the eye, inner ear, spinal cord, and the brain. It also allows the reattachment of

185

amputatd fingers, and the suturing of minute nerves and blood vessels as well as the reversal of vasectomies. This type of procedure, although very small-scale, uses the familiar "open surgery" method.

Minimally invasive surgery, known popularly as "keyhole surgery", entails the performance of surgical procedures using an operating laparoscope or endoscope (an optical device for viewing inside the body), which is passed though a tiny incision. The operating instruments are also passed, and operated through similar small incisions (entry ports). Such methods usually allow the patient to resume normal activity much sooner than with conventional procedures. There is also less visible scarring.

Whilst laparoscopic (entry into the abdomen) procedures have been performed for over 50 years, the early endeavours were cumbersome and difficult to manage, since the surgeon had to operate, using the endoscope in one hand, and a single instrument in the other. During the late 1980s several developments took place which helped to improve the scope of endoscopic surgery. These included the development of sterilisable high-resolution video-cameras, the appearance of a new generation of surgical telescopes with wide angle lenses, and the provision of halogen high intensity light sources operating with fibre-optic connections. These improvements allowed the use of a video link, which gave every member of the operating team the chance to view the procedure on a large screen, while allowing the surgeon to use both hands.

The next significant advance was the development, mainly in France and the US, of a range of versatile miniature instruments capable of performing all the movements and actions required in a conventional surgical operation. It should be mentioned here that in endoscopic operations, working space is created by inflating the cavity with carbon dioxide gas. The development of specialised access ports fitted with valves, made it easier to maintain the inflation pressure.

Minimally invasive surgery, or minimal access surgery, may be said to have its serious beginnings in the removal (in France 1988) of a patient's gall bladder (cholecsystectomy). The procedure is now used in almost every case where surgical intervention is needed, to obtain access to the interior of the body, either for observation, removal or repair. It will be sufficient here to give examples of two important fields of medicine: cardiovascular interventions, and cancer research.

10.2.1. Cardiovascular Intervention

In conventional bypass surgery a blood vessel, taken from the leg or chest, is grafted between the aorta, and a point in the coronary artery beyond a narrowing or blockage. The graft will then require stitching, taking up to ten minutes. Keyhole surgery, through a small hole in the chest, despite its advantages for the patient, makes it more difficult to sew the graft into place. Also, since patients are usually given anticoagulant drugs, there is the chance of leakage for some time after the operation.

A new device developed by Tony Anson of Anson Medical, and tested by Professor Gianni Angelini, of the Bristol Heart Institute, UK, (1), uses a small plastic connector which is held in place using a hose clip made from a memory metal (see Chapter 9). The graft is shown in Fig. 10.1, and the ultimate intention is that all the components should be assembled in one catheter, which could cut the artery, deploy the device, pull out the branch, make the connection and seal it with the hose clip. Because the device is housed within the artery, it is not necessary to use immunosuppressive or anticoagulant drugs, and the insertion can be undertaken while the heart and lungs continue to work normally.

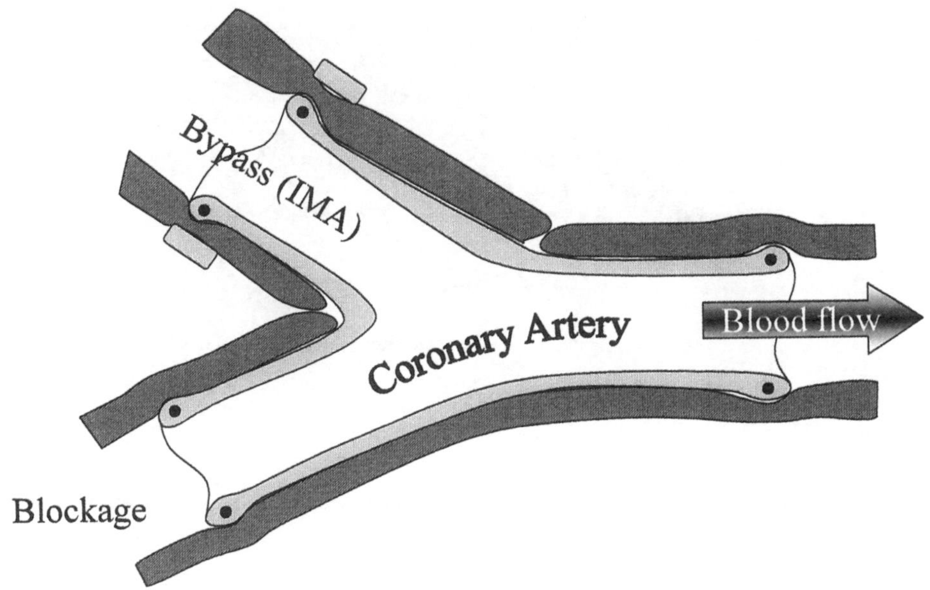

Figure 10.1 The sutureless arterial graft, (Courtesy Anson Medical & Department of Health)

10.2.2. Cancer Research

Over 85% of breast cancers are said to develop in the multitude of tiny milk ducts which spread out from the nipple. Unfortunately this is one of the most inaccessible parts of the body, and by the time the X-rays used in screening tests are able to detect cancers, they may have been growing for years.

Surgeons in Guy's Hospital, London realised that what was required was a tiny probe which could see into these ducts in order to detect the early stages of cancer. A team led by Dr Nicholas Beechey-Newman enlisted the aid of film technicians from Hollywood, who were expert in the use of fibre optics to create special 3-D effects. By modifying the lighting system and improving the quality of the image, they produced an endoscope as thin as a human hair, which could be inserted, under local anaesthetic, into the nipple. Once inside, coloured images were projected onto a video screen, so that doctors could detect tissue changes. Normal healthy tissue looks like smooth white tubes, while cancerous ducts are red and blocked.

This revolutionary new technique is already being used on patients, with considerable success (2). Fig.10.2 shows the probe and ancillary equipment.

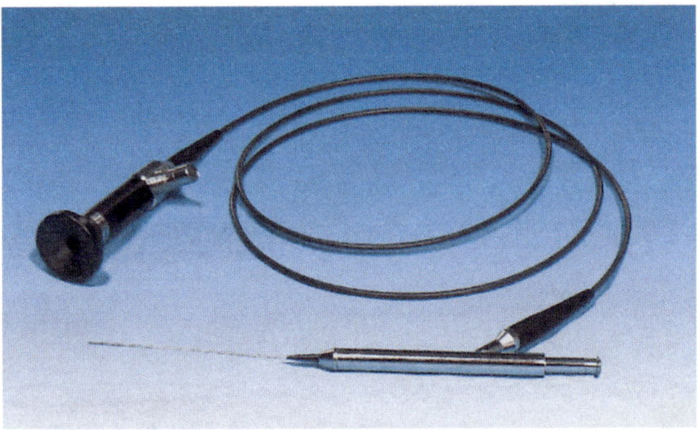

Figure 10.2 The ultra small camera probe for breast cancer screening (Courtesy Nicholas Beechey-Newman, Guys Hospital, London)

10.3. The Coming of Robotics

The use of robotics, long the dream of science fiction writers, has been commonplace in industry for many years, notably on car assembly lines and for complex machining operations. It is also employed wherever it is necessary to avoid contamination of, or by, sensitive materials; for example in the nuclear power industry, or in biological research.

It is the very repetitiveness of the tasks undertaken by robots, the need to perform a series of frequently highly complex operations with a high degree of precision, over and over again, that makes the use of robots cost-effective. It is when we try to give robots comparatively mundane and boring tasks, such as acting as porters, or carrying medications around hospital wards, that the concept fails; they cannot cope with the everyday uncertainties of life. For instance, in the mid 1990s, Northwick Park Hospital in Middlesex, England, experimented with a robot porter called Jeeves (what else?). After only a few months the project had to be abandoned because it couldn't handle the unexpected hazards, ranging from closed doors to patients who thought it was a mobile cash machine!

It is in the operating theatre, however, that the robot really comes into its own. Guided by computer-generated 3-D images, robots are able to wield scalpels and other surgical tools with far greater accuracy than a human surgeon. In addition, they are not distracted, don't get tired or ill, or have to cancel operations. They also have infinitely steadier hands than any of their human counterparts.

One of the earliest successes of robotics was in orthopaedic surgery. Operations, such as total or partial hip replacements, involve a considerable amount of sawing, drilling, chiselling and hammering. The surgeon has to cut a channel in the femur to fit the shank of the replacement joint, and this may require several attempts before a perfect fit is achieved. Robots can perform the necessary cutting with great precision, using a template generated by magnetic resonance imaging (MRI) scanning techniques. A device called "Robodoc" was developed for this purpose, in 1992, by a Californian company, Integrated Surgical Systems (ISS). The set-up consists of two elements:

* A planning station – on which the surgeon can match the joint to the bone dimensions, and so determine how much bone needs to be removed
* A mechanical arm – which is placed in position once the surgeon has made an incision and exposed the site of the operation.

The use of teleoperating systems, together with virtual environment—the fusion of robotics and three-dimensional imaging technology—allow the control of a laparoscopic camera (an endoscope with a viewing tube and camera attachment) to be undertaken while the surgeon operates; also assisted by robots.

Voice activation of a surgical robotic assistant has made possible single-surgeon thoracic surgery (3). The surgeon registers voice commands into a voice card, and the thorascope is connected to a robotic arm.

The teleoperating systems and telesurgery permit the operator to perform surgery from a remote site, using a three-dimensional camera fitted with tactile, auditory and proprioceptive feedback, (a proprioceptor is a specialised sensory nerve-ending that monitors internal changes in the body brought about by movement and muscular activity). This technology may provide a means to treat patients in hazardous or distant environments where evacuation is not feasible. NASA has a programme to develop such procedures for the proposed manned 3-year mission to Mars, which will follow the un-manned forays in 2004..

It is evident that the advent and exploitation of robotics in the operating theatre, far from making the surgeon superfluous, will require a team of highly trained and skilled individuals. It provides also an interesting mix of materials: the robot itself, while largely constructed of metal, contains many plastics parts. It is also, to keep it sterile, swathed in disposable polyethylene sheets, as to some extent are those of the surgical team who are in the operating theatre. The use of robotic surgery has so much potential for the future, that I believe it would be helpful to include several different views of the disposition of the people and instruments, as well as the general layout and types of equipment in modern robotic operating theatres. Fig. 10.3(a) shows a plan view of the theatre supplied by the University of Pennsylvania Medical Center.

(a)

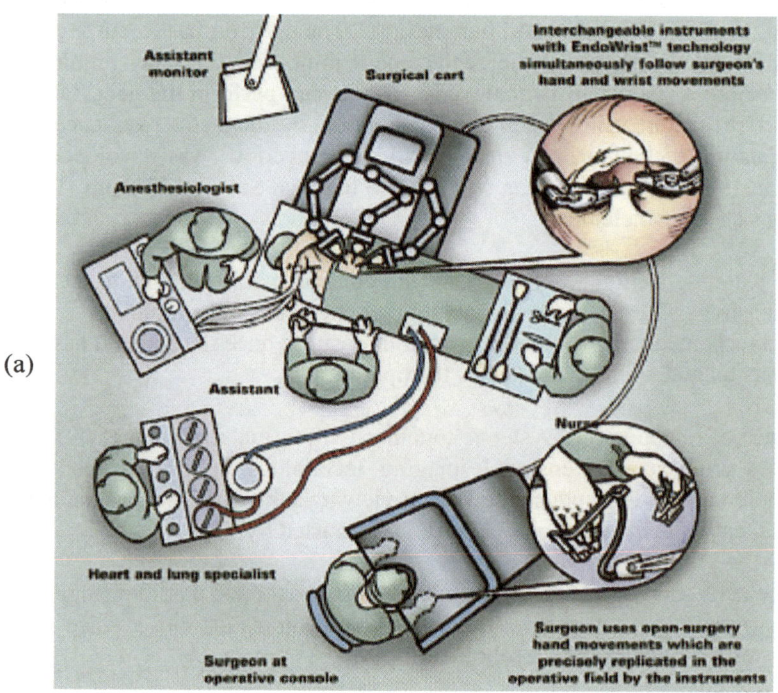

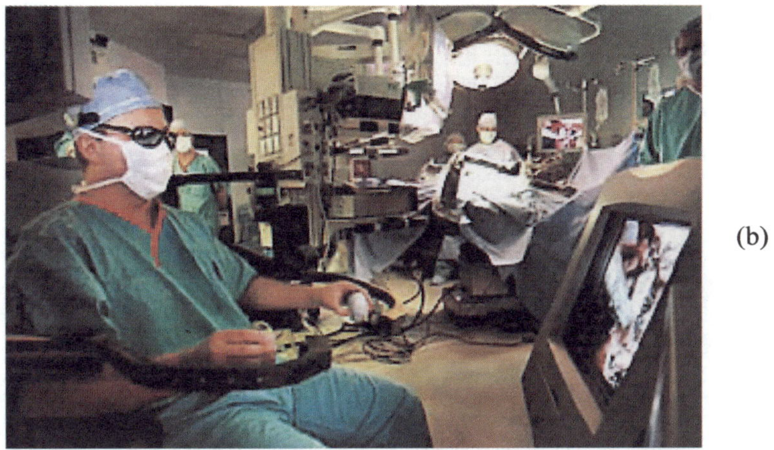

(b)

(c)

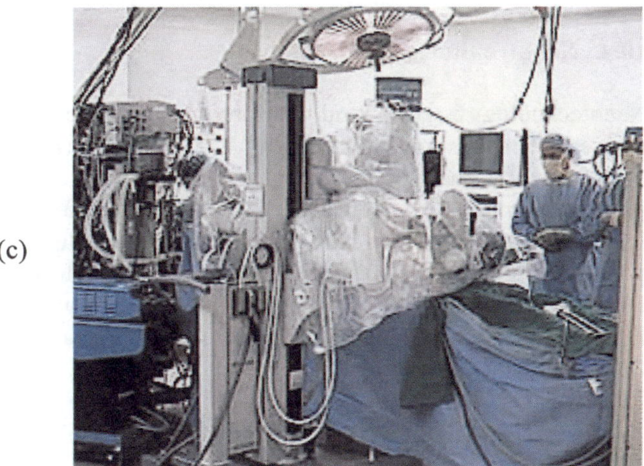

Fig. 10.3(b) shows the surgeon operating the robotic controls while seated in front of a video screen; other assistants are in the background. Fig. 10.3(c) illustrates an operating theatre which contains the "da Vinci" robotic system, and Fig. 10.3(d) (overleaf) shows surgeons at St Mary's Hospital, London, performing a prostate operation with the "da Vinci" set-up. The system has three robotic arms, operated by the surgeon using joysticks. The arms are inserted into the body through an opening little more than 1 cm across, and the surgeon gets a three-dimensional image of the

course of the operation through two tiny cameras mounted on one of the arms. Precision is essential, particularly in prostate surgery, since the gland lies close to nerves which control the bladder, and the sexual function. This type of surgery also requires a high degree of skill on the part of the surgeon, since the instruments have to be accurately positioned in order to pass them through the small opening.

(d) 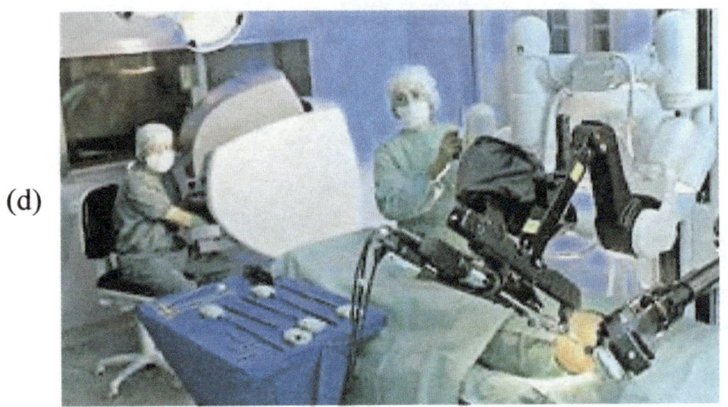

Figure 10.3 Views of modern "robotic" operating theatres

10.4. Nanotechnology

Nanotechnology is concerned with products and events which take place in a world whose dimensions range from about $10^{-8} - 10^{-10}$ m (roughly one thousand millionth of a metre!). Since many scientists believe that some of the most far-reaching discoveries in the next decade are likely to come from work in this field, particularly in the interaction between man-made and natural materials, we need to appreciate the size of existing products and processes. Fig. 10.4 illustrates how some familiar, and some not so familiar, objects appear on a scale from 10 to 10^{-10} metres. Once this has been grasped, we can discuss some of the materials and techniques that are currently under development.

10.4.1. Spider Silk

Among the most interesting and complex examples in this category of materials is "spider silk". Web building spiders produce a variety of fibrous silks, exhibiting properties ranging from Kevlar-like fibres with three times the tensile strength of mild steel, to rubber-like elastomers. This diversity of properties is what gives the finished web its essential characteristics: the strong radial fibres serve primarily as scaffolding to support the structure, while the "capture" zone—made from loosely coiled spirals—absorbs the energy of a flying insect, without damaging the web.

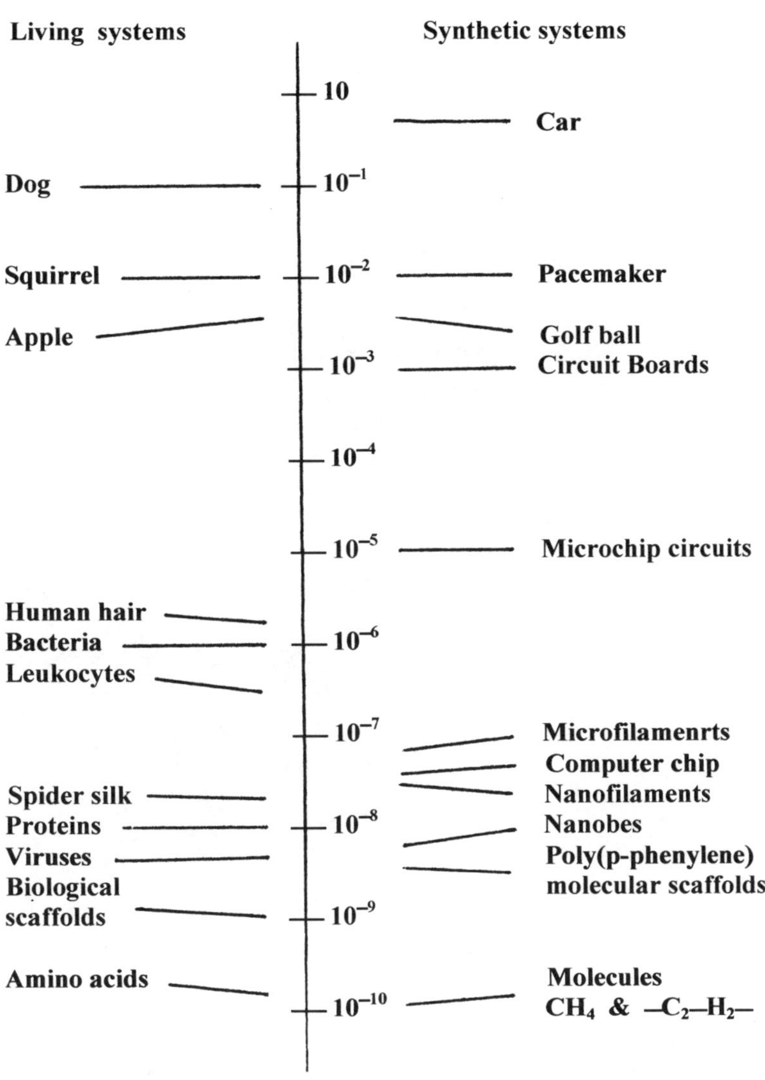

Figure 10.4 A size comparison of some familiar, and not so familiar, objects

Spider silk has been known, and handled, for many millions of years—indeed, it has recently been reported (4) that the earliest known sample has been found preserved in Lebanese amber, and that it is more than 120 million years old.

However, it is only recently that its chemical structure and properties have been properly understood, and consequently—because of its potential for a number of exciting applications—many researchers have jumped on the bandwagon.

Spider silk is composed largely of a polymerised protein called fibroine, and is extruded from the silk glands (spigots) on the body of the insect   Fig. 10.5 shows the anatomy of the spider, and a view of the glands from which the silk emerges

(a)

(b)

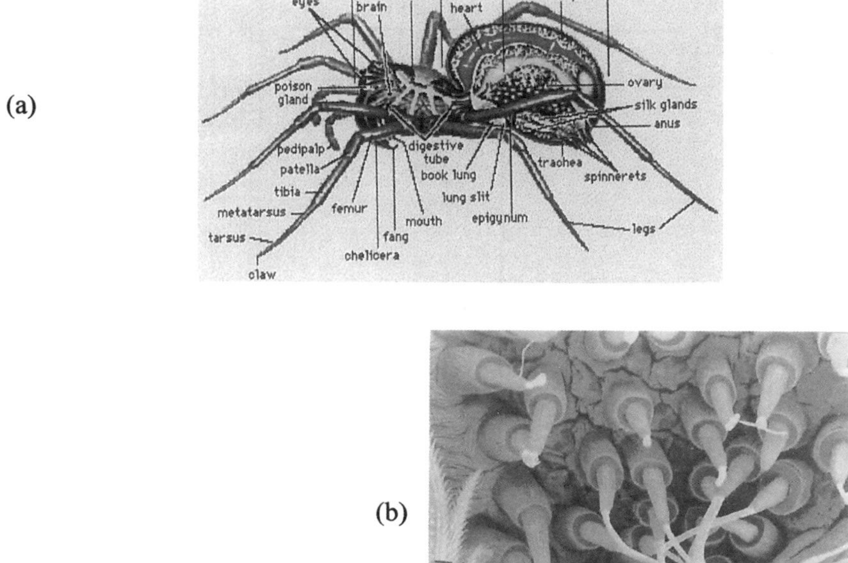

Figure 10.5 (a) Side view of the spider showing the silk glands (b) an enlarged view of the same glands (spigots)

In its natural unstretched state, the silk exists as a series of chains of loosely coiled molecules, some 200,000 – 300,000 links in length. Whilst experiments have been carried out with spider silk as a potential suture material, the variability of supply, and lack of consistency oof the natural material has proved a major impediment. However, an exciting new development, pioneered by Nexia Biotechnologies Inc. and the US Army, has resulted in the production of a novel synthetic fibre (BioSteel) 5 times as strong as steel (5).

The process consists in extracting the silk-producing gene from a golden orb weaver spider, and inserting it into a fertilised goat's egg. The egg is then implanted into a host mother, whose offspring will produce milk containing complex proteins, which are then treated and forced through spigots, giving a spider silk type polymer.

Possible applications so far considered include extra light body armour, biodegradable fishing lines, medical sutures, and scaffolding for cell culture. An interesting idea, recently described in the New Scientist (6), has resulted in the production of hollow optical fibres only 1 micrometre in diameter. Yushan Yan, and a team from the University of California, dip-coated short lengths of fibre with tetraethyl orthosilicate, and—after drying—baked them to burn away the silk, leaving hollow silica tubes.

If the planned objective of producing tubes with cores less than 10 nanometres in diameter is achieved, they could replace the relatively limited carbon nanotubes currently used to study supramolecular chemistry; a world in which reaction rates become speeded up and matter behaves differently. Fibres could also be used for ultra-small microscopes, which would not cause damage to the sample in the way an electron microscope does.

10.4.2. Artificial Muscles

There are many articulated devices, including: artificial limbs, remote sensing probes, small space vehicles, aircraft servo-control systems &c, where the present method of operation, electric and pneumatic motors, springs and levers, is perfectly acceptable. However, the provision of a device which approximates more closely to the natural human muscle is a more complex challenge, because its creation and operation will need to call upon the resources of the polymer chemist, the physicist, the medical scientist, and the engineer.

The role of such a device, although not all in the same one at the same time, would be replacement of the function of diseased or paralysed muscles in the body, power to the articulation of limb prostheses, and—because space technology is so often the source of so many ingenious systems—the provision of a means of "moving, gripping and lifting" for small space robots, such as the one shown in Fig. 10.6. This small palm-sized rover contains optical and infrared instruments, whose viewing windows are kept clear of dust by miniature "windscreen wipers" made from lightweight polymer, and made to travel backwads and forwards by the application of electric currents.

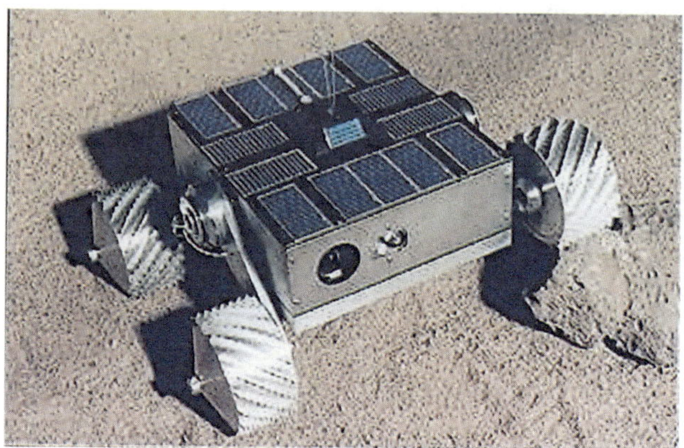

Figure 10.6 The NASA nanorover destined to explore an asteroid

Flexible polymer ribbons made from chains of carbon, fluorine and oxygen molecules, respond to an electric current by the movement of the charged particles (ions) in the polymer. Depending on the polarity (–ve or +ve charge) on the ribbon's two sides, it will be pushed or pulled into a new shape. Four such ribbons have been fabricated into a gripper for the rover, which is capable of picking up samples (see Fig. 10.7).

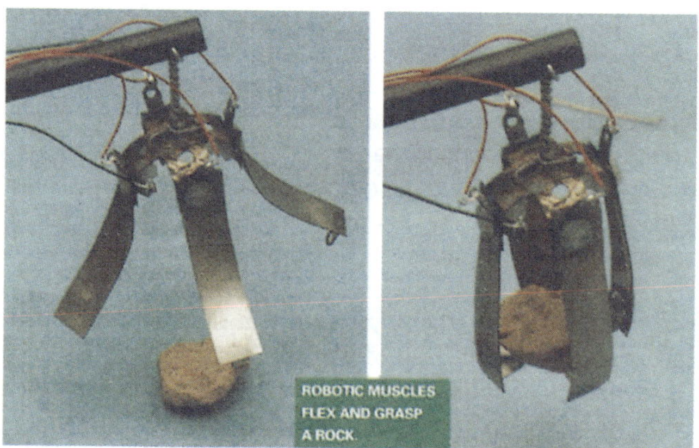

Figure 10.7 A gripper fabricated from strips of EAP (Courtesy NASA, Jet Propulsion Laboratory)

Since it is known that normal muscles are activated by small electrical charges generated by the brain, some encouraging research has been carried out on the stimulation of paralysed leg and arm muscles by the application of external electric currents through electrodes implanted in the wasted muscles (7). An example of this technique is given later in this chapter.

More recently attention has focussed on the behaviour of certain types of polymer, which react to different stimuli. At the University of New Mexico, Professor Mohsen Shahinpoor and his team have developed artificial muscles from polyacrylonitrile, a substance that is a combination of a gel and a polymer, which changes its shape when its pH (acidity) is altered (8). He also believes that a band of artificial muscle, attached to the eyeball, could be activated by a small electromagnet so as to change the shape of the eye and bring blurred images into focus (9). The operation of the device is shown schematically in Fig. 10.8.

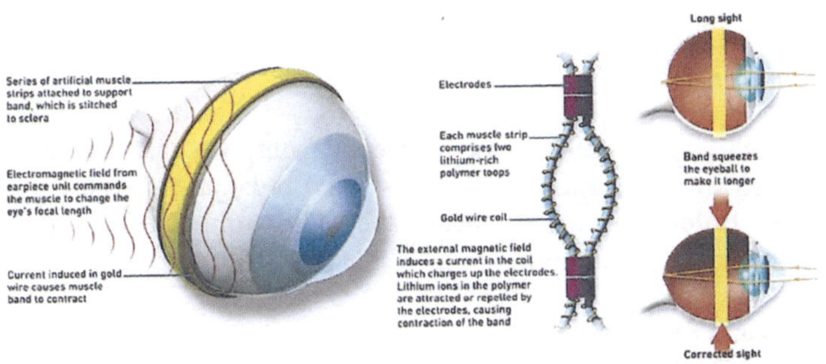

Figure 10.8 The use of artificial muscles in the correction of poor sight (Courtesy Professor Mohsen Shahinpoor, University of New Mexico)

10.4.3. *Nanobes and Nanofilaments*

It will have been noted that, in Fig. 10.4, I have placed a family of polymeric substances called nanobes and nanofilaments on the right, or synthetic, side of the picture. This is partly to avoid cluttering up the other side, which is already well filled, and partly because researchers are not entirely sure if they are living or synthetic. Whatever they are, nanobe colonies were discovered in Australia in 1998 by Dr Philippa Uwins (10), and were found to contain the elements carbon, oxygen and nitrogen. When their properties are more clearly understood, it is possible that they may have a role to play in medicine (11).

Readers will have observed that I have used the word "exciting" many times in this book, and I make no apology for so doing, for I believe that, in particular, the world of nanotechnology, linking as it does both natural and synthetic materials on a molecular scale, is one of the fields in which the most exciting discoveries are likely to be made.

10.5. A Look into the Future — A Miscellany of Technologies

I think it is appropriate to end this book with a brief look towards the future. In the main part of the work I have attempted to cover the essential surgical techniques, the materials which are used in them, as well as to highlight some of the areas which are ripe for development. Let us now consider some which offer such a compelling case that they must influence the pattern of medical and surgical advances in the future.

10.5.1. General Considerations

If we look over the whole field of medical endeavour, we can see that there are certain requirements in the design of techniques and prostheses that are universal in their importance. It does not matter whether they apply to machines or devices, and they may be summarised as follows:

* Lightness and Smallness
* Precision and Reproducibility
* Biocompatiblity – matching the behaviour of natural materials
* Reliability – or at least the ability to repair and replace rapidly
* Versatility – the ability to utilise unusual sources of power such as the brain
* Sophistication – breaking down the barriers between the natural and synthetic

What follows are some examples, which have emerged during the preparation of this book as topics of the future. It must be appreciated in all this however, that there are certain forces at work, which do not all pull in the same direction, leading inevitably to compromises in what can be achieved, and what is appropriate. These include:

* The wellbeing of the patient
* A justification of the need for such equipment
* A comparison of the cost of having it, compared with the use of simpler, cheaper and, perhaps, more effective techniques.
* Ethical considerations – whether or not such procedures are "morally right"

10.5.2. *Harnessing the Mind*

When, in Chapter 2, we considered the increasing sophistication of modern artificial limbs, we also thought about the next stage: using the electrical impulses generated by the brain to power machines. Considerable research has been carried out with monkeys, but my former colleague at Reading University, England—Professor Kevin Warwick, of the Department of Cybernetics—has carried the concept a stage further, by having an electronic pickup (a sophisticated microchip) surgically implanted into a nerve in his arm; enabling him to be plugged directly into a computer By this means he is able to perform a variety of tasks at a distance, including operating a prosthetic hand. (see Fig.10.9). Warwick's work, and the thinking behind it is contained in his book " I, Cyborg" (12).

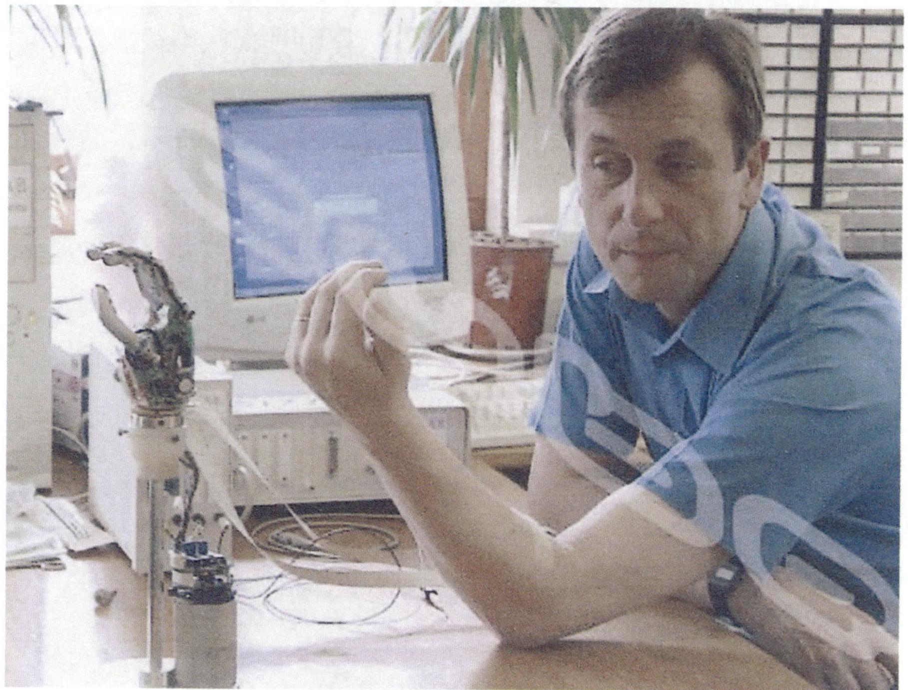

Figure 10.9 Professor Kevin Warwick and the bionic arm

Another example of the use of technology to promote the use of paralysed muscles and nerves, is that carried out on a tetraplegic by John Hobby, Consultant Surgeon at the Spinal Unit, Salisbury Hospital, England. Pioneered in the USA, the technique—known as the "Freehand System"— entailed the implantation of 8 small electrodes on the muscles in the right hand and arm.

These electrodes are connected to a small receiver and stimulator, implanted into the muscle just below the collarbone. Signals are received from a transmitter coil on the chest, connected to a small computer attached to the user's wheelchair. Muscles and tendons were taken from other parts of the body to reinforce and strengthen the operation of the arm and hand, which was initiated by movement of the shoulder. So successful is the procedure, that the patient is contemplating having the same done to the left arm, next year. A schematic view of the procedure is shown in Fig. 10.10.

(a)

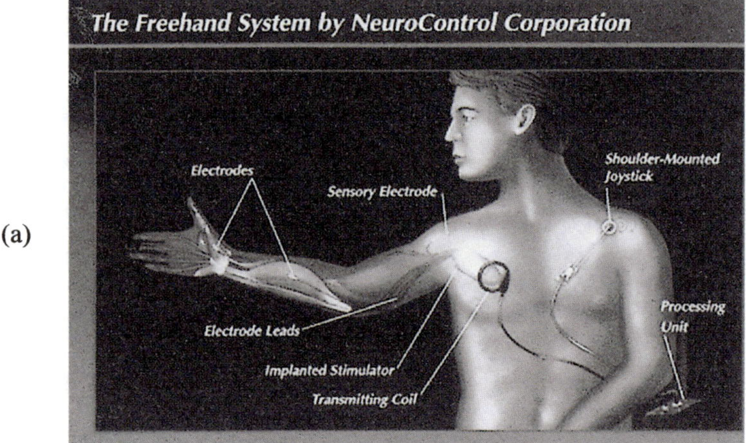

(b)

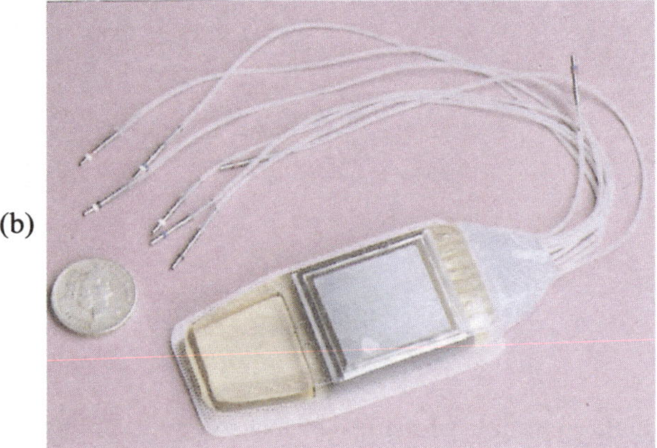

Figure 10.10 Illustration of (a) the circuitry devised to allow movement of a paralysed arm and hand (b) the implantable device (Courtesy J Hobby & P Taylor, Spinal Unit, Salisbury Hospital, UK, and the Neuro Control Corporation, USA)))

Another device which uses electrical stimulation, is that developed at the Catholic University of Louvain (13). The "artificial eye" provokes visual sensations in the brain by directly stimulating different parts of the optic nerve. Fig. 10.11 gives an illustration of the basic principles of the device.

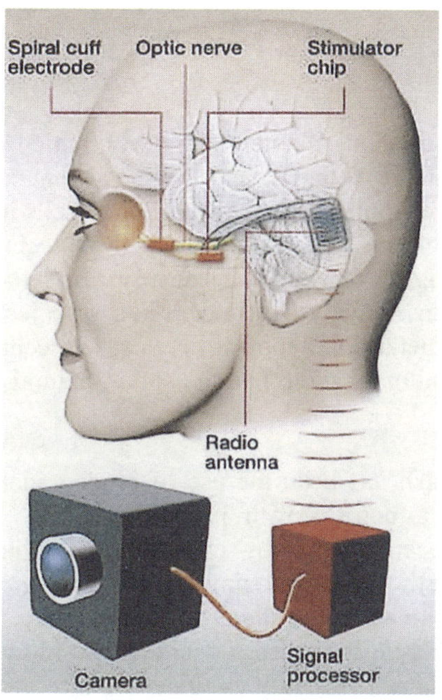

Figure 10.11   The restoration of sight by stimulating the optic nerve (Courtesy The New Scientist)

Although both complex and costly these techniques have been studied in several countries, and have brought new life and mobility to people with paralysed limbs and damaged eyes. The next stage could be in the development of implantable devices which are capable of stimulating the brain into producing the necessary signals, in much the same way as the pacemaker does for the heart.

Encouraging though these inventions are, and they will undoubtedly be developed to the stage where they can safely help many people, the real goal surely must be to develop materials that can be used to replace damaged nerves and muscles, and which work as nearly as possible in the same way as the "real thing". As we saw earlier, within the last few years, several research centres have set up programmes of work to study the development of muscle fibres made from synthetic polymers, as well as the possible application of the so-called "memory materials", both polymers and metals. Notable among them is the Artificial Muscle Research Institute, Albuquerque, New Mexico, USA. These endeavours are certainly showing promising results. However, in a closely allied field, directed towards the same goal, advances are being made in the development of "biopolymers" grown from muscle and nerve stem cells.

10.5.3. New Materials

We have already noted in previous chapters that the ceramic hydroxyapatite, applied as a coating to an implanted prosthesis, and the metal tantalum—in the form of a sintered cage—are able to encourage the growth of bone cells in orthopaedic surgery, and in the reconstruction of jaw defects.   Both of these techniques, however, have the disadvantage of leaving a "foreign" substance in the body, which might—at a later stage—cause problems either of disintegration, or rejection.   Also the very strength and rigidity of a metal bone implant may cause mechanical stress problems by being much stronger and more rigid than the softer, natural materials surrounding it.

A more recent approach has been the use of biodegradable polymer scaffolds which contain grains of a bone growth promoting agent.   Three-dimensional polymer scaffolds have been created by cross-linking collagen conjugated with hyaluronan (poly-L-lactide). These are similar to the materials we considered in Chapter 6 when dealing with sutures. The resulting structure, in which small grains of hydroxyapatite are anchored, is shaped by conventional low temperature polymer processing techniques, and has the ability to adhere both to hard and soft tissue. As the scaffold is resorbed into the body, and fully metabolised (therefore harmless), bone cells form round the hydroyxapatite.

A whole range of new biomaterials and techniques is surveyed in an excellent series of articles by Jon Katz, from which I will only refer to one.   I propose now to select only one other example of this type of technology.   This is the use of combinatorial and supramolecular chemistry. In the former case, a relatively small number of ingredients is assembled together under carefully controlled conditions to produce a "library" of biomaterials, each with its own specific range of properties.

Supramolecular chemistry is concerned with the development of molecular assemblies for biological applications which mimic the nature and performance of natural nanomaterials (we have already discussed the general principles of nanotechnology earlier in this chapter). As an illustration we can cite the behaviour of polyrotaxanes. These are molecules comprising cyclic components threaded onto linear chains capped with bulky end groups; shown schematically in Fig. 10.12.   In one case, the cyclic components were found to migrate towards one end of the chain as the temperature was increased. This molecular piston mimics the action found in natural tissue contractions.

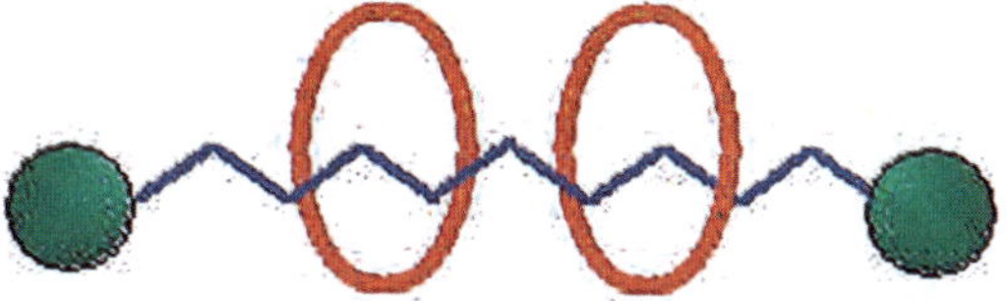

Figure 10.12 Example of a polyrotaxane supramolecular polymer structure

Another potential use for such "smart" materials is in the controlled delivery of insulin for the treatment of diabetes. The system features an insulin-containing porous membrane made from a copolymer {poly(methacrylic acid-g-poly[ethylene glycol])}containing glucose oxidase. The surface of the membrane contains a series of molecular "gates" which open to release insulin when the interaction between the glucose oxidase and the glucose in the body reaches a critical level. The process is illustrated diagrammatically in Fig. 10.13.

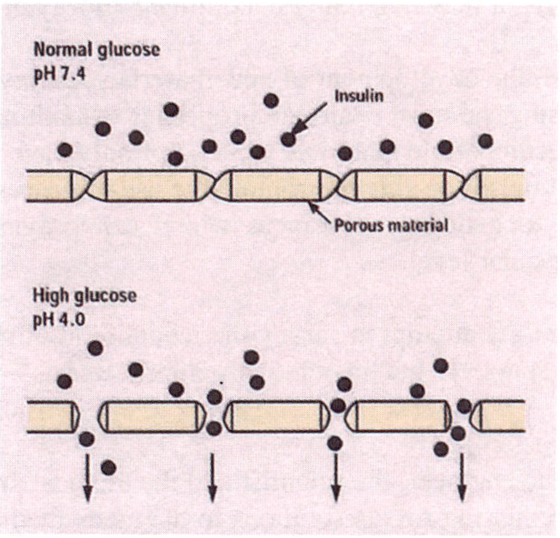

Figure 10.13 A hydrogel insulin delivery system (Courtesy Jon Katz)

My final example, announced in December 2003, is the development by a research team at Ohio University—led by Douglas Goetz, of biodegradable polymer particles which mimic white blood cells (15).

The bead, which is made of polygalactic acid and polyethylene glycol—and coated with the appropriate targeting molecules—can not only travel to the site of a bacterial infection, or wound, but also to the site of tissue inflammation. White cells (leukocytes) can do the former, but—faced with an inflammation caused by eg arthritis, heart disease, or inflammatory bowel disease—they tend to migrate to areas where they aren't needed, and cause further damage.

10.6. Conclusion

It will be evident from this very brief survey of new ideas and technologies, many of them extremely ingenious and complex, that the whole field of medicine and surgery has reached an important and critical crossroads where far-reaching decisions have to be made.

On the one hand we have the ever-increasing miniaturisation, and consequent complexity, of surgical techniques, which—since they enter and leave the body with decreasing delay and damage—must be beneficial. What we have to balance this against, though, is the increasing cost of providing and operating the equipment, as well as the need to recruit and train new surgical teams. It seems likely, too that these factors will lead to the establishment of a network of very expensive "centres of excellence", which may, or may not, really benefit the majority of patients.

On the other hand, the development of new materials has revealed a tremendous opportunity for accessing the most desirable properties of both natural and synthetic polymers to create biocompatible materials which, not only have a minimal effect on the immune system, but also are able to promote the use of processes such as cloning and gene technology to generate substances which can provide tools capable of functioning at the molecular level.

Finally, I hope that my attempt to survey the whole field of medical and surgical endeavour—however sparsely, but in relatively simple terms—will have achieved three things at least:

* To show how the engineer, the scientist and the medical practitioner can, and must, work together to provide solutions to the many medical problems which still exist
* To communicate some of the excitement which I have gained from working in so rewarding a field
* To made the reader want to know more about the subject.

If I have managed to do so, I shall be well satisfied.

References

(1) Anson T., *Maintaining vascularity by optimisationn of haemodynamics in a novel sutureless anastomosis device,* "Challenges in Biomaterials" (2003), 28 March.

(2) Beechey-Newman N., Guy's Hospital, (2002).

(3) Schaaf T R., *Robotic Surgery: The Future Is Now, Medical Devicelink,* (2001), March

(4) Zschokke S., *Nature,* **424,** (2003), 636–7.

(5) Turner J., *et al.,* Nexia Biotechnologies Inc.,& US Army (2002)

(6) Yushan Yan, *New Scientist,* (2003), 19 March.

(7) Hobby J., Spinal Unit, Salisbury Hospital, UK, (2001).

(8) Shahinpoor M., University of New Mexico, Report, (2001).

(9) Shahinpoor M., *New Scientist,* (2002), 21 March.

(10) Uwins P., *American Mineralogist,* **83,** (1998), 1541–1550

(11) Selleh A., *Space & Astronomy,* (2001, 19 December.

(12) Warwick K., *I, Cyborg,* (Century, London, 2002)

(13) Veraart C., *New Scientist,* (2000), 29 April.

(14) Katz J., *J Smart Mateials,* **10,** (2001), 819–833

(15) Gibson A., *EurekAlert (Athens, Ohio),* (2003), 17 December)

FURTHER READING

For those who are interested in following up some of the topices touched upon in this book, I have given a short list of recent book titles. I have not read most of them, but—from the reviews—they appear to be well recommended. I have also found it useful to search the internet for review articles on specific topics by government agencies, university departments or medical schools.

Surgery

Kremer K., ed., *Atlas of Operative Surgery:Surgical Anatomy, Indicaions, Techniques, Complications: Minimally Invasive Abdominal Surgery* (Thieme Publishng Goup, 2001)

Baumgartner William A., et al., *Atlas of Cardiac Surgery* (Hanley & Belfus Inc., 2000)

Kirklin J W. and Barratt-Boyes Brian G., *Cardiac Surgery* (Churchill Livingstone, 2003)

Clements F. and Shanewise J., *Minimally Invasive Cardiac & Vascular Surgery Techniques* (Lippincott Williams & Wilkins, 2001)

Lattimore C R., *Key Topics in General Surgery* (BIOS Scientfic Publishers Inc., 2002)

Cushieri Sir A., et al., *Essential Surgical Practices* (Butterworth-Heineman, 14th Edition)

Biomaterials

Park J B., *Biomaterials: Principles & Applications* (Interpharma/CRC, 2002)

Wise D L., ed., *Biomaterials in Orthopaedics* (Marcel Dekker Inc., 2003(

Palsson B., ed., *Tissue Engineering* (Prentice-Hall, 2003)

Combe E., *Dental Biomaterials* (Kluwer Academic Publishers, 1999)

Prokop A., ed., *Bioartificial Organs* (New York Academy of Sciences, 1998)

Dumitriow S., ed., *Polymeric Biomaterials* (Marcel Dekker Inc., 2001)

Nanotechnology

Owens F J., *Introduction to Nanotechnology: Selected Topics* (John Wiley & Sons Inc., 2003)

Wilson M. And Smith G., *Nanotechnology: Basic Science & Emerging Technologies* (Interpharma/CRC 2002)

Nalwa H S., ed., *Encyclopaedia of Nanotechnology* (American Scientific Publishers, 2004)

SUBJECT INDEX

A

Abdominal surgery, 3, *see* Aneurysm
Acrylic polymers, *see* polymethyl meth-
acrylate (PMMA)
Adhesion, prevention, 120
Alloys, non-magnetic, 135
Aluminium, 45, 58, 59, 77, 109
Anaesthetics/Anaesthesia
  methods, 3, 4
  types of, 3, 4
Analgesia, 3, 4
Aneurysm, repair of, 8, 16, 17, 18
Angioplasty, 90, 91, 92
Ankle, *see* Othopaedic surgery
Arteries, narrowed, 19, 90
  repair of, 8, 9
  see Heart Surgey
  see also Vascular surgery
Artificial heart, *see* Mechanical heart
Artificial heart valves, 125–131
  mechanical, 126, 127, 128
  tissue, 114, 128, 129, 130, 131

B

Biocompatiblity (also Bioacceptability),
63, 67–70, 73, 75, 77, 79, 80, 82, 83, 87,
94, 102, 103, 105, 113, 117, 119, 120,
122, 126, 128, 129, 131,132, 135, 137,
139, 146–49, 155, 156, 159, 167, 169,
187, 198, 202, 203
Blood
  clotting mechanism, 66, 67
  composition, 6, 64, 65
  damage, 64, 97, 102, 126
  dialysis, 94–101
  groups, 6
  transfusion, 5
Blood oxygenator, 101–105
  membranes, 103–104
  tubes/hollow fibres, 104, 105
Bone
  behaviour, 151

damage, 151–153, 157, 158, 160, 162
167
growth/ingrowth, 68, 122, 126, 138,
141, 146–148, 150, 155, 156
Brain, *see* Neurosurgery
Brass, 32
Bronze, 44, 170, 172, 176
Burns, 73–**75**

C

Carbon fibres, *see* Reinforced materials
Carbon, 29, 30, 31, 33, 166, 181
  pyrolytic, 128, 131
Cardiac Surgery, 8–16, 18, 186
  see also Heart Surgery
Cardiac bypass equipment, *see* Blood
oxygenator
Cardiac assist devices, 131–136
  defibrillators, 136
  pacemakers, 131–135
Catheters, 85–90
Cellulose, 94, 95
Ceramics, 34–36, 68, 113, 153, 155,
159, 167, 169, 172, 195
  see also Hydroxyapatite
Chromium, *see* Steel
Cobalt, *see* Steel
Contact lenses, 78–83
  flexible, 78–83
  rigid, 78, 79, 81
Copper, 32, 44, 159, 172
Cosmetic surgery, 136–141, 149
  breast implants, 136–141
  other areas & reconstruction, 141, 149
Cotton, 75, 77, 116
Crystal
  structure, 30–32
  dislocations, 32

D

Dacron, *see* Polyester
Defibrillators, *see* Cardiac assist devices
Dentistry, 141–150